Hypnotherapy: An Alternative Path to Health and Happiness

Hypnotherapy: An Alternative Path to Health and Happiness

To Mary Courtney,

Blessings for a
brand new life of
Health & Happiness!

Kweethai Neill

Kweethai Chin Neill, PhD

9-5-2014

Library of Congress Control Number: 2007910025
ISBN: Hardcover   978-0-9816385-0-8
               Softcover   978-0-09816385-1-5

This book was printed in the United States of America.

To order additional copies of this book, contact:

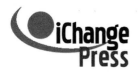

1-817-491-9809
www.ihealththerapies.com

CONTENTS

Introduction: University to Universe-city 19
    Transition..19
    The hook...20
    New commitment 21
    iHealth model of integrated wellness 24
    Graduate school 24
    Boyned! 25
    Double rainbow...26
    Home to Texas 27

Chapter One: Dump the myths.....................................29
    Quack like a duck?..29
    What *is* hypnosis?..30

Chapter Two: Hypnosis Primer....................................33
    Natural, relaxing, and healthy....................................33
    Open to suggestion..34
    Control 34
    Consent, not ability 34
    Heightened acuity...35
    Time 35
    Split time/space 35
    Abreaction 36
    Mind knows, brain shows..36

Chapter Three: Hypnosis and consciousness 37
    Mind, Brain, or Consciousness?................................37
    Spectrum of consciousness 39
    Trance is natural 41
    Stop thinking 42

Everyday trance 43
   Road trance...43
   Movie trance 44
   Book trance..44
   Advertisement trance 45
Subconscious Notebook 46

Chapter Four: Applications for hypnosis.....................47
   Hypnosis in action 47
      Magic show 47
      Self-hypnotism 49
      Hypnotherapy...52
   Hypnotherapy vs. self-hypnosis 53
   Choice and Consent 54

Chapter Five: Path to health and happiness................55
   Health vs. Suffering 55
   Investment in suffering 56
   Mental expectation 56
   Choose not to choose is a choice 60
   Coping 62
   Genesis of suffering 62

Chapter Six: Energy of fear 67
   Fundamental fears 67
   Degrees of fear..68

Chapter Seven: Choose to heal....................................71
   Be exceptional 71
   I'm good enough! 73
   Time to change...74
   Give up a blessing to receive a blessing 75
   White pill effect...76

Chapter Eight: Hypnotherapy is health care 79
    Health care or medical care? 79
    More health care, please 85

Chapter Nine: Alternative path to health 89
    Alternative or complementary medicine? 89
    Trust takes courage 90
    Healing to be whole 92

Chapter Ten: A spiritual experience 93
    Spiritual or religious? 93
    Gardener for your soul 96

Chapter Eleven: Hypnotherapy Highlights....................................97
    Alternative medicine 97
    Natural medicine 98
    Spiritual healing 98
    Restorative power 99
    Effective and fast 100
    To be recovered 100

Chapter Twelve: Characteristics of hypnotherapy.......................101
    Why rather than What and How...................................101
    Who can benefit? 103
    Necessary dispositions...105
    Desire to change 105
    Willingness to focus...107
    No more alibis 108
    Courage to take action 109
    Trying is lying..110

Chapter Thirteen: Hypnotherapy is transforming.......................113
    Discover your subconscious..113
    A formative practice 115

Chapter Fourteen: Hypnotherapist as professional.......................119
    Bona fide profession...119
    Caveat emptor..121
    Who can be a hypnotherapist?.................................121

Chapter Fifteen: Fundamentals of hypnotherapy.....................123
    Making change happen...123
    Analysis based on Model of Change 125
    Changing long-held beliefs 128
    Upgrade the software 130
    Reboot the subconscious 131

Chapter Sixteen: Mechanics of hypnotherapy 133
    Hypnotherapy step-by-step..133
        Trust the hypnotherapist....................................133
        Integrate responsibility and response-ability........133
        Spiritual work..134
        Energy work 135
        Suggestibility is willingness 136
        Relaxation routine..137
        Promotion of healing 139
        Reflection and reinforcement 141

Chapter Seventeen: Power of language and intentions 143
    Start right now! 143
    Personal energy work...144
    Genesis of mental expectations.................................145
    Elephants, pain, and weight.....................................145
    Power of words..148
    Cup half empty or half full? 149
    Manifesting intentions 150

Epilogue...153
Checklist..155
Bibliography 157
A Set of Brief Comments/Summaries 165
About the Author 169

DEDICATION

To my best friend, colleague, companion, and soul mate, Dr. Steve Stork; without your left hand, my right hand could not possibly have turned out this work. Thank you for your boundless faith in me, in my work, and in this book. Thank you for your saintly patience and profound guidance in editing this book. My cup runneth over with gratitude, respect, and love.

FOREWORD

By Gil Boyne

This is the first in what I suspect will be a significant series of books by this author. I first met Kweethai Neill as a member of a master class I was teaching. I immediately noticed her excitement and expressiveness. It was clear to me she was developing a full realization of the power of hypnosis and its many applications in therapeutic practice.

She brings to hypnotherapy an impressive background as a university professor and health educator. As a seasoned professor, her presence in any master class, either as student or teacher, typically results in stimulating discussions and better understanding for all persons involved. That, indeed, is what she also brings to this book.

Dr. Neill has created a clear, comprehensive, and diverse overview of hypnotherapy suitable to anyone seeking to comprehend modern hypnotherapy as an alternative to more traditional, allopathic medicine. While that serves aspiring hypnotherapists well, it also presents her unique take on the subject.

Professor Neill brings rich life experience to bear in this book and in her practice of hypnotherapy. A brief biography of her academic background segues into her discovery of hypnotherapy as an alternative career choice, and her subsequent immersion in the teaching and practice of it.

The result is a well written, lucid, and well organized treatment that bridges the gap between hypnotic technique and clinical intervention. The clarity with which she describes the uses of hypnotherapy is helpful to anyone either contemplating it for themselves or exploring the field as a career alternative. Also, since the writing is often directed at the reader as someone contemplating hypnotherapy, the book provides practicing hypnotherapists with explicit rationales to support its value and usefulness.

I recommend this book to anyone wishing to learn more about hypnotherapy, and to those who wish to improve their skills using hypnosis in a therapeutic practice. Extending a long tradition, Dr. Kweethai Neill shows that putting a client in trance is the easy part; knowing what to do once they're in trance is where the therapy really happens.

PREFACE

When I left the university, I had no idea what I would do next. I only knew that I had to leave what I was doing. Later, when I chose to become a hypnotherapist, I wondered how I could use my academic experience as a teacher and researcher to enhance my practice.

I am a health educator. I remained a health educator even as I began to practice hypnotherapy. Only, I am now more effective. This new tool helps people really *change* their behaviors to become healthier or happier. There is no greater excitement for me than helping people get on with their lives, some experiencing joy for the first time in their life.

In the years I taught at the university, I felt successful when students "got it," demonstrating that they understood the purpose of health promotion. It was thrilling to see a spark of passion light up in them. I see that same excitement every day now as I work with clients. Only today, that spark is the light of spirits being rekindled as they reconnect with themselves.

There are many books that describe and attempt to explain hypnotherapy. I have read many of them. So why another one? What makes this book distinctive? I came to hypnotherapy while following a path of inquiry I hoped would lead to a new way of looking at health promotion. What I found remains as surprising to me as to anyone who knew me during my years as an academic. My conclusion is that most of the theories that guide health education and health promotion are well-intentioned, but not very effective. And though some of those theories are usually quite complex, the real answers are amazingly simple, and the simple answers work best!

After exploring an array of alternative health modalities, I chose to become a clinical hypnotherapist. Along the way, I developed a process I now call Integrative Hypnotherapy (IHT). It is a composite of the knowledge and skills accumulated during my career as a health educator. I summarize that process in this book, saving the details for another book in which I can do better justice to them. The focus of this book is basic hypnotherapy.

Hypnotherapy can help you attain a better state of health and happiness. Surprisingly, it's a rather simple process. But some of the simplest things in life seem the hardest to accept. This book will help you understand the basic rationale, so you can fully invest yourself in the process should you seek the services of a hypnotherapist.

I will explain how hypnosis is used to help reframe subconscious programs that prevent you from being healthier and happier. If you already have a good life, congratulations! Read on to find out how you can turn a good life into a great life. If there are aspects of your life you desire to change, this book will give you tools with which to plan and get the help necessary to implement those changes.

Hypnosis has been used in many cultures, and for centuries, in religious rituals, in healing traditions, and in modern-day advertising and marketing. For many, the words *hypnosis*, *trance*, and *hypnotherapy* conjure up mysterious misunderstandings that cause them to be afraid. Some people fear even being near someone who practices trance induction, let alone becoming hypnosis subjects.

Misassumptions about hypnosis commonly begin with, "Will you make me cluck like a chicken or quack like a duck?" In stage hypnotism, the subject appears to be at the mercy of the hypnotist, often being made to do silly things for an audience who eagerly anticipates being entertained. This book unravels the myths that stop many from considering how hypnosis can be used for healing. Understanding those myths would allow them not only to openly engage in hypnosis for self-empowerment, but to share their experience with others.

Can you imagine sitting through a root canal without anesthesia? Can you imagine giving birth with no pain? How about giving up smoking or alcohol without the use of pins or pills? How about losing weight without suffering the rigors of dieting? Imagine getting over stuttering after only a few sessions with a hypnotherapist? It sounds too good to be true, doesn't it?

The anesthetic effects of hypnosis serve utilitarian purposes while reducing exposure to potentially harmful chemicals or medications. In contrast, addictions—whether to toxic substances or toxic relationships, or even to maladaptive behaviors and habits—are really forms of self-betrayal that require deeper probing. Hypnotherapy can help disengage the fear that perpetuates negativity; turning it into self-love. This creates a spiritual transformation that opens the door for you to be all you can be. What are you waiting for? Are you ready to find out about hypnotherapy?

Self-hypnosis is a simple tool that can help you take charge of your own health and happiness, whether or not you desire therapy. You can choose to be better than you currently are. Why settle for *good* when *great* is available?

The solution is simple; the choice is yours. Health and happiness is only as far away as a twinkle of an eye. If you need help, hypnotherapy is available, whether you choose to try it as your own hypnotist (in self-hypnosis) or seek the help of a trained professional (as in engaging a certified clinical hypnotherapist). Hypnotherapy is an alternative path to health and happiness. I have seen it work time and time again, and now you can also. Are you ready to find out?

ACKNOWLEDGEMENTS

I am who I am today because of the generous kindness of my teachers. Teachers mold us by guiding, coaching, challenging, and facilitating our process. As I learn to be a teacher, I learn to be a better student. I want to honor and give thanks to those who have taught me formally or touched me by their love and support in academia; in particular, Drs. Diane Allensworth and Tom Dinero, and Dr. Tom Kordinak and Dr. Chwee Lye Chng and Carol Hummel, valued friends and mentors. I also honor those who have taught me in less formal institutions: Grandmaster Lin Yun, Dr. Carol Bridges, Donna Eden, Ormond McGill, Joey Korn, Bette Epstein. Their work and guidance have influenced me to change. I also thank all my clients, students, and readers, who continue to teach me every day in the university that has no walls, my Universe-city. I honor my parents, who gave me their wisdom, unconditionally coated with love and faith. Deep gratitude to my beloved brother, the late Dr. Chin Kwei Cheong, who nurtured my spirit to be the best I can be. I give thanks to my children, who challenge me to grow, no matter how painful. To my many teachers, and especially to Gil Boyne, my father in hypnotherapy; I *kowtow* (bow on my knees and with head on the ground) in gratitude. To my students past and present, clients, colleagues, friends, and now you, my readers; please don't stop challenging me to new heights. Thank you for picking up this book and walking this path with me.

Kweethai Chin Neill, PhD, CHT, CHES, FASHA

INTRODUCTION

University to Universe-city

Transition

I resigned as department chair at a prominent university, a move that closed the door to my career in academia. I should have been very scared. I had invested several years of hard work to get my doctorate. Yet I was bidding a fond farewell to additional years of teaching, doing research, writing grants, publishing research papers, presenting at professional conferences. I enjoyed those activities and was sad to leave them behind. Most of all, I would miss my students. I would miss the sparkle in their eyes as they transitioned from backpacks to briefcases. I would miss sitting in my regalia at graduation, praying for them as they received their diploma. I would also miss the hugs. Most were a thank-you from students for structuring my classes in ways that helped them make important choices to change their lifestyle habits.

But there were other things I wouldn't miss. University faculty find themselves sitting through hours and hours of futile meetings. Too many department meetings I attended consisted of lengthy discussions that accomplished little more than covering sloppy errors and negotiating reduced responsibilities. As department chair, my main responsibility was seemingly to complete reams of meaningless reports. And the joy of teaching was dampened by the agony of evaluations (both of me and by me). Rather than being scared, I experienced an incredulous sense of liberation!

I am a teacher. All I ever wanted to do is to teach. Spending time pushing paper that went nowhere did not resonate with my soul. Taking on the role of department chair was a choice spawned from ego—rising to the top—that, as it turns out, was inconsistent with the mission of my work. While many academic administrators thrive in their work, it was wrong for me. Leaving the university was not only a logical choice, it was a soulful decision. Strangely, as it dawned on me that the decision was final, I felt not fear but a profound sense of calm. It felt good; I felt free.

I resigned without any prospects. There was no new job awaiting, and I had no clue what to do next. Yet I was not afraid. I was more concerned that I was not concerned; within a few months I would have no paycheck. But I was free!

The hook

The Universe moved me into a new realm, away from academia into . . . what? . . . I had no idea . . . yet. As a gesture to my newfound freedom, since I no longer needed to work on weekends, I attended a dowsing conference in Dallas. I had taken a course in dowsing as part of some prior training in feng shui (the Chinese science of environmental design). My friend and dowsing teacher, Joey Korn, was teaching at the conference, and I attended to show my support.

On a rainy morning the day after the conference, I returned to Dallas to pick up Jill, Joey's wife, to show her around town while Joey taught a postconference workshop. Jill and Joey were staying at Bette Epstein's house, the woman who had organized the conference. Jill was not ready when I arrived. I've wondered since if that could have been divine intervention. I ended up having a very nice conversation with Bette.

I discovered Bette was a hypnotherapist. "Hypno-what?" I was fascinated. I knew what hypnosis was, but this was the first time it had come up in conversation this way. My curiosity was immediately piqued. "So," I asked, "how did you get started in it?"

When Bette was a teenager, she and her sister saw a stage hypnotist perform. Bette's sister, though painfully shy, allowed herself to be hypnotized and was given the confidence to deliver a speech. Bette was fascinated to witness her usually reticent sister speak with flawless confidence. This led her to understand the body can be made to do what you want it to via a direct suggestion.

Many years later, Bette was out on a routine fitness run. It was raining. She slipped and fell onto the curb of the road, hitting her face in the process. She was badly hurt and bleeding freely. She was at least a mile from home, with no one to help her. As she lay on the wet pavement, she remembered the hypnotist and decided to try hypnosis. She gave herself a direct suggestion to stop bleeding and for the pain to stop. Somehow, she was able to get herself home. Her husband immediately saw how badly Bette's face was injured and called his friend, a plastic surgeon, to meet them at the emergency room. After hours of surgery, Bette was restored. According to the surgeon, her face had been badly lacerated, but she presented at the hospital with no active bleeding. Bette healed miraculously and with few scars.

"Wait, Bette, you mean you actually can tell your body to stop bleeding?"

"Yes, that was what I did. And now I teach hypnotherapy."

I was hooked. "Tell me more!" I found out later there is so much more you can do with hypnosis. I started to read about the subject. When I found out that Bette was offering a class that summer, I went to study with her and never looked back.

New commitment

I was so sure of my eventual success in this new endeavor that, one week before taking the exam to become a clinical hypnotherapist, I bought an office property. But neither did I leave anything to chance.

In my first three years of practice, I studied with every expert in the field I could find. I am fortunate to have had many illustrious teachers, among them Ormond McGill and Gil Boyne (who I dubbed "the Wizard of Hypnotherapy"). I built a library of literature on hypnosis and hypnotherapy. I also started reading about energy medicine. It was a fast and furious adventure to new knowledge. The universe plunged me into a new school—my own Universe-city!

I studied with Donna Eden and Dr. Barbara Brennan in energy medicine. It made sense to me to expand my quest into this new science. It follows from the work I had been doing in health literacy; which had previously led me to study feng shui. For the prior five years, I had been engaged in a personal research project, studying how to create harmonious spaces. Harmonious living spaces can enhance your health, and I thought such spaces would also make people more comfortable communicating with their doctor.

Dr. Carol Bridges reintroduced me to my spiritual heritage through her shamanic style of feng shui practice. Joey Korn taught me about the Kabbalah and energy dowsing. Then, studying with Grandmaster Lin Yun (who is credited with bringing feng shui to America) was a culminating experience. These were the professors of my new Universe-city.

Somehow, gathering this new knowledge made me value my existing education even more. I was inspired to integrate the new into what I had learned from my professors and teachers in health behaviors and health promotion. Not neglecting my education professors who had taught me how to teach or how my law school professors had explained people and the law. I found all sorts of new folks who had important lessons in life to teach me. It's been exhilarating, spinning in a cosmic soup of reclaimed energies.

While busy learning and practicing, I also learned the importance of stilling myself enough to listen to my own spirit. Ultimately, the way I practice the art of hypnotherapy evolved into a unique style. I weaved into the process all that I picked up about human behavior and everything I was discovering about energy medicine. The result is a model of practice that presents to each client an individualized tapestry of wisdom, knowledge, and skills synthesized through my experiences as a health educator, researcher, scholar, and, most importantly, as a survivor of my own healing journey in Life. I still promote health, but now I promote healthy spirit, mind, and body; putting spirit first in the mind-body-spirit paradigm.

Many years ago, while teaching a course on the Foundations of Health Education, I constructed a definition for my students. "The goal of a health educator is to inform, teach, motivate, inspire, persuade, and to facilitate individuals, families, and communities to consciously engage in behaviors that will help them live healthier and happier lives." In other words, the goal of the health educator, my goal, is to help people *change* behaviors to be healthy and happy. It is a challenging goal. Behavior change was hardly obvious among my university students. I suspected most would experience similar resistance to their own efforts to promote change as they became health educators themselves.

The most uncomfortable aspect of leaving the university was the thought that I might also be giving up on health education. Yet I discovered much in common between what I had been teaching and what I was preparing to practice. My search had led to a new way to express my passion for helping people become healthy (health promotion) and happy (hypnotherapy). I remain a health educator. Only now I can more effectively influence change. The combination of health promotion and hypnotherapy does a more complete job of helping individuals become entirely healthy, inside and out—mind, body, and spirit.

I use my skills as a hypnotherapist to help people get unstuck, setting their spirit free. After that, I teach them how to sustain this newfound freedom by training and coaching them in healthy behaviors and healthy communication (Life Enhancement Training). Last, but not least, I apply the principles of feng shui to help them design and create physical and social environments that are supportive and appropriate for this healthier and happier persona.

Eureka! I call this innovation the iHealth Model. I call the process Integrative Hypnotherapy (IHT). The IHT process applies Clinical

Hypnotherapy, Life Enhancement Training, and feng shui to help people be in harmony with themselves, to connect with God and with the environment.

In weaving this tapestry, I found a new home for my passion. I launched, as a recovered academic, from the university into a new career as a scientist in the Universe-city of Life.

iHealth model of integrated wellness

The iHealth model is the simplest way to express what I do as a health educator. The "i" in iHealth has several meanings. First, it represents *integrated*, or whole, including wellness within mind, body, and spirit. Second, it represents the *individual*; you have to take responsibility for personal change. Third, the "i" is in lowercase. When you have attained the life you desire, you change from a lowercase "i" to a capital "I." The capital "I" represents the power of the Universe, or God. When your individual divinity is aligned with the Universal Cosmos, or God—or, when you find the holiness within your own spirit and understand that it is connected with the divinity of the Universe, or God—you are healthy. IHT empowers you toward that type of change. Change brings healing. And healing makes you whole again. The idea of wholeness resides within the word *health*. To be *healthy* means to be *healed* or *whole*. To have "iHealth" means to be healthy and happy, inside and out.

Graduate school

Having embarked in my new universe for learning, there has been no turning back. Teachers show up in my life in many forms. Some are found in regular classrooms, and the rest hold forth in the classroom with no boundaries. The person who has most influenced my practice of hypnotherapy is Gil Boyne, a giant in every aspect. Boyne's book, *Transforming Therapy*, was one of the first I read in my new quest for knowledge in hypnotherapy. I had also seen videotapes of his work. His technique of instant induction stirred my curiosity. There was a certain powerful energy about him that I found refreshing, though some people find it intimidating. I felt a certain powerful connection with this man although we had never met. So off I went to see the Wizard, the Wizard of Hypnotherapy!

Boyned!

There is a Zen Buddhist saying, "When the student is ready, the teacher appears!" I signed up for Gil Boyne's master class. For five days, I was totally taken over by Boyne. At eighty-two years old, the man commanded the room like a warrior in his thirties. Never mind that he had to use a cane—the result of recent knee surgery—his vitality pervaded. Over five, continuous days, Boyne dazzled his students with passionate teaching. His case stories, arising from fifty-two years of experience in the field, were invaluable. I tumbled head-over-heels in love. Here's my next mentor! I was smitten. I was entirely intoxicated by Boyne's delivery, the passionate energy he exuded about hypnotherapy, and his generous desire to impart on his students everything and anything he knew about hypnotherapy.

His classroom management style was commanding and authoritative, but always respectful and sensitive. Throughout, he taught with precision and compassion. There was never any doubt he was in charge. (You had better not be late coming back from a break!)

I learned that this characteristic of taking charge is necessary for effective *transforming therapy*. There was something about his fearlessness that resonated with me. I was exhilarated to watch the master at work. By the fifth day, I could no longer contain my excitement. I went to Boyne and asked if I might have a conversation with him. He graciously agreed and told me to wait till he found a moment. The master class ended, and a conference accompanying it commenced. I waited . . . and waited. After a few days, Boyne finally set a time and place. I was to wait for him at his book table. I had hoped for a few minutes of chat, but we ended up talking for two and a half hours. It felt like we were old friends from another time. I expressed my excitement about him and his work. Feeling a patriotic obligation to preserve a national treasure, I offered to write down his stories. It was surprising to hear the words flowing out like verbal diarrhea. Yet I was thinking to myself, "Boyne is a national treasure of knowledge, skills, experience, and wisdom, and I must do something to ensure that his work and passion for this profession is preserved and shared." I offered to write his biography.

I also wanted him to be my mentor. I formally asked, "Gil, will you be my mentor?" With a twinkle in his eye, he said, "Will you *marry* me?" In that instant, in the presence of God and witnessed by mutual respect, we were connected intellectually and spiritually.

Double rainbow

A buzz of creative energy surged in me after my conversation with Boyne. I had a new teacher. And not just any teacher, but someone willing to be my mentor as well. I immediately cancelled a study series with another teacher. I could study with her later. After all, she was sixty years old, while Boyne was eighty-two. I had no idea what would happen next with Boyne, but I *knew* I must clear my slate to be available. The universe always provides. Returning to my office from the conference, I received an invitation to deliver a seminar in Albuquerque. It was on one of the dates I had just cleared. I was thrilled because Santa Fe, where Boyne lives, is only an hour's drive away. I called Boyne and offered to visit if he would consent.

He did. With no agenda, I spent a few days simply conversing with Gil Boyne. I left Santa Fe after four days, carrying with me about twenty-four hours of recorded conversations. Most precious to me was Gil's friendship and the trust he placed in me by sharing many personal stories. Many were recorded to be used in future books. Others were off-the-record and will never be repeated. For four days, we got started around nine in the morning and sometimes did not stop until nine at night. I was thirty years younger than Gil, but found myself running to keep up. What a phenomenon!

The afternoon I drove back from Santa Fe back to Albuquerque, the rain had just stopped and the air was filled with freshness. My soul thrilled at being launched into a sea of creative energies. Mountains escorted me most of the way, but looking past them, I saw a double rainbow. That pair of rainbows followed me all the way to Albuquerque. I wondered, Is this a sign?

The conversations with Gil convinced me I had found my niche. I became totally committed, rekindling the fire in my belly. Answering the call from my soul had led me to a new vocation. Hypnotherapists don't retire. There is no need to. When you love what you do, it's not *work*, meaning there's nothing to retire *from*. As of this writing, Boyne remains fully active. Ormond McGill, another leading figure in hypnotherapy, taught right up until the week he died at age ninety-two.

In subsequent conversations with Gil, I mentioned I wanted to start a school for hypnotherapists. He suggested Dallas as a good location. He didn't know my grandchild would soon be born there. That could be no accident. At the time, I was practicing in Georgia. My husband was a university professor; but he readily agreed to join me in the Universe-city.

Home to Texas

With passionate commitment and wholehearted excitement, I relocated to Texas. My mission is to teach all I know to anyone who seeks to learn about the wonders of hypnotherapy and the powers of self-leadership. I am excited to share all I know in helping you attain **iHealth.** I do this individually in private sessions and collectively in seminars. Further, I train others who are interested in embarking on a career in hypnotherapy through courses in my school.

I hope this book whets your appetite for learning how to empower yourself with the *response-ability* for your own life and happiness. I hope to help you create an *ability-to-respond* to all the wonderful gifts God has bestowed on you. All you have to do is to be still, look, listen, learn, and embrace life. Life is good if you wish it. Life is *great* if you *want* it. What do you choose?

CHAPTER ONE

Dump the myths

Quack like a duck?

Many folks have different ideas of what hypnosis is. While some people are intrigued by it, it scares others; though neither group knows exactly why. Have you ever experienced hypnosis? Have you seen it on TV or watched a hypnosis show on stage? The lack of direct experience with hypnosis has resulted in many popular myths and untruths about it. At the very least, hypnosis is considered an unnatural state since it is so rarely experienced—and then only under the guidance of a *hypnotist* (who is also regarded with curiosity, if not suspicion). At the worst, hypnosis is associated with mind control, voodoo, perhaps even the work of the devil. These, too, are misconceptions.

Most people incorrectly equate hypnosis with sleep, the only difference being that under hypnosis you comply with suggestions to do things you normally wouldn't do. In fact, the term *hypnosis* is derived from Hypnos, the Greek god of sleep. Often, a person in hypnotic trance appears to be asleep (eyes closed, body relaxed). The term *hypnosis* was coined to describe this sleeplike condition. Hypnosis is, in reality, a state of consciousness quite distinct from sleep. So equating *hypnosis* with sleep is incorrect.

What misconceptions do you harbor? Do you imagine being hypnotized to waddle around quacking like a duck, as in a stage show? Or do you imagine a man with an *evil eye* putting you to sleep and ordering you to do bad things you are powerless to resist, as in the movies? If so, it's understandable that hypnosis might scare you. After all, Svengali-type characters are quite intimidating! You would be right to be concerned that you might be made to do things against your will.

But these are misconceptions and myths. The assumption that you can be made to commit acts against your will or beliefs has been perpetuated by books and movies that depict unscrupulous schemers using hypnosis to direct unwitting dupes to commit crimes in their behalf. It makes for an interesting screenplay, but people generally cannot be hypnotized to commit crimes or other immoral acts. The scenario is simply not feasible in real life. Movies exaggerate mysterious phenomena for dramatic effect. It leads you to misconceive them as true. They are *not*.

There are, of course, circumstances under which subjects are asked—in the context of a stage show—to do things they would normally find embarrassing or even impossible, but those things are limited to fun and entertainment. Hypnosis cannot make you do something you consider immoral or unethical. There is no need to fear hypnotism. Read on to find out more about hypnosis. The knowledge will set you free from your apprehensions. There really is nothing to fear.

What *is* hypnosis?

Hypnosis takes a variety of forms, several of which I describe in this book. The basic definition in the Webster dictionary is:

> *Hyp.no.sis: 1. a state that resembles sleep but is induced by a hypnotizer whose suggestions are readily accepted by the subject.*
> *2. any of various conditions that resemble sleep*

In most literature, *hypnosis* is used interchangeably with *hypnotism* to refer to the act of inducing hypnosis. To improve clarity within this text, I refer to *hypnotism* as either the study of hypnosis or the act of inducing hypnosis and to *hypnosis* as being in the state of trance. Hence, *self-hypnotism* describes the act of inducing trance on yourself, and *self-hypnosis* is the trance state you then experience. Yes, that means you can serve as both hypnotist and subject. That's only one of the many wonders of hypnotherapy!

Hypnotherapy is a process in which trained professionals engage hypnotism to remove old ideas and replace them with new suggestions. This helps clients who are experiencing challenging life situations to get unstuck. The purpose of training clients in self-hypnosis is to support changes introduced during the formal hypnotherapy sessions.

No one knows exactly how hypnosis works. But we know this much. *Hypnosis* is a natural state of consciousness in which your awareness is heightened while your cognition rests. Some call this a state of trance. In this state of mind, you are most open to suggestions made directly to your subconscious.

At this point, you may be curious to know what it feels like to be hypnotized. I can't tell you any more than I can describe what it's like to hold a moonbeam in your hand. Just as, though I've experienced it twice with excruciating clarity, I don't have the eloquence to describe the sensations of childbirth. These are uniquely personal experiences. You have to actually go through the process yourself to adequately understand. Male doctors, though they may deliver hundreds of babies, are still voyeurs of the childbirth process. They will never know what it is like to feel a delivery on a firsthand basis. Anyone who has experienced hypnosis can try to describe, explain, or define it, but the map is not the territory. Try it and you will then know what I mean.

CHAPTER TWO

Hypnosis Primer

Natural, relaxing, and healthy

According to Gil Boyne, founder of the American Council of Hypnotist Examiners, hypnosis is a natural state of mind characterized by specific traits. When in trance, you experience an extraordinary quality of mental, physical, and emotional relaxation. This is an extraordinary sensation, one that is only brought about in hypnosis. This sensation is unique to hypnosis because the quality of relaxation is different from sleep or drug-induced states of mind.

Hypnosis is a *natural state of consciousness*. The experience is pleasant and enjoyable, and when used appropriately can be an effective therapeutic tool. The adjective *natural* means there is no need to use artificial means, such as drugs or special devices, to induce a hypnotic state. It happens naturally as sleep although hypnosis is *not* sleep. The focus is on the word *natural*.

Natural also means that any healthy individual is capable of experiencing hypnosis—as naturally as they experience falling asleep or having a dream. *Natural* means there are no ill side effects. You return to full awareness after trance, feeling relaxed and refreshed. No drug can offer that.

Open to suggestion

During hypnosis, you are increasingly open to suggestions of new behaviors. You are emotionally driven to act on suggestions, directions, or instructions given by the hypnotist. You experience a strong motivation to perform that behavior. Why does this happen? During trance, your cognitive brain takes a rest from analytical and critical functions. That allows the subconscious to take over. It accepts new information less critically. The subconscious is like early computers that lacked spelling and grammar checkers; whatever data you type in, it accepts without discrimination. In trance, you are more ready to take in instructions and accept directions.

Control

This openness to suggestions may be disconcerting to you right now, if you've never experienced a hypnotic state. But remember, you will only comply if the suggestions are consistent with your own moral compass. Nothing will happen if the directions conflict with your desires or your beliefs. There is still that element of will and consent that belongs only to you. Therefore, if you really do not want to quack like a duck, you won't; but if you don't mind quacking like a duck, you will when the hypnotist suggests that you do. On the other hand, for example, if you really do not want to quit smoking, no degree of trance can make you quit. You are still in full control of all your actions.

Consent, not *ability*

You see, trance work is not about whether or not you *can* be hypnotized, it is about whether or not you **want** to be hypnotized. Unless you have an organic dysfunction of the brain or you are heavily medicated, if you can carry on a wakeful conversation, you have the capacity to go into trance. That is, if you wish to. It is clearly a matter of whether you *want* to be hypnotized, not if you *can* be hypnotized.

Heightened acuity

While hypnotized, you experience a heightened sense of awareness. You feel that you hear better and *see* more clearly. You feel an increased capacity for taste, smell, and touch as well. Clients often give me very detailed descriptions of their hypnotic travels (trance-travel). They can *smell* the cookies baking in their grandmother's kitchen or describe the vibrant colors of flowers in a garden they find themselves in. They even *feel* the exact emotions of situations evoked within trance.

You experience the events as if you were actually there, even more clearly than you might in everyday wakefulness. This is one of the features of trance that forensic hypnotists employ to help witnesses remember crime scenes.

Time

When you are in trance, time takes on a whole different meaning. You may feel as if a few minutes had lapsed when in fact an hour has passed in real time. This is very common in my office. You are surprised how "quickly" time passes. You return to your usual wakefulness to discover that two hours have gone by, when it feels like mere minutes.

Split time/space

You feel as if you are in two places at once. For example, you may experience the acute sensations of walking on the beach in your imagination, so vividly you can feel the sand between your toes, smell the sea and taste the ocean salt in the air, yet you are still aware of being in the room with the hypnotist.

Abreaction

You may even take on a new persona as you fully enter the role of your trance-imagination while simultaneously explaining the experience to the hypnotherapist. Sometimes you may speak differently, or in another language. Going back to a time in your childhood, you may speak like a child while still communicating with your hypnotist as an adult. You'll also likely feel the same emotions of the event more intensely than you can remember (abreaction). Often at this point, healing occurs as the skilled hypnotherapist guides you to resolve the issues.

Mind knows, brain shows

Many skeptics insist on empirical data to show that hypnosis exists. Hypnosis is just another status of your sense of awareness or consciousness. The advent of the electroencephalogram (EEG) has allowed scientists to measure brain activity, to identify various "states of consciousness." When fully conscious, brain activity registers at more than 14 cycles per second (14-32 cps, *beta state*) on the EEG. As you prepare to go to sleep, the brain slows down. In the dreamy state just before you fall completely asleep, or just prior to fully waking in the morning, brain activity slows to 7-14 cps, *alpha state*. This is the realm of the subconscious mind, a state where you daydream or experience REM (rapid eye movement) sleep. As brain activity slows even further to 4-7 cps, *theta state*, subliminal conditioning can take place. Most hypnotic trance occurs in the alpha state. Some deeper trance work, such as past life regression, is conducted when brain activity is in the theta state. As the brain slows to less than 4 cps, *delta state*, you become unconscious. Of course, brain activity stops at 0 cps—you are legally dead. Biofeedback procedures often use this type of measurement to show how busy your brain is.

CHAPTER THREE

Hypnosis and consciousness

Mind, Brain, or Consciousness?

The *brain* is an organ with billions of nerve cells. Those cells process information and send out messages, activating responses to external stimuli. Modern science depicts the *mind* as the sum total of all the cellular activity within the brain. That makes *consciousness* an expression of the *mind-brain connection*. However, emerging evidence suggests that *consciousness* is more a product of cellular activity occurring throughout the body, not just in the brain. In other words, consciousness is more expansive than just the mind. In fact, energy medicine suggests that consciousness is not even limited to the body.

Rather, there is a nonphysical, *psychic* if you will, dimension to consciousness. Ormond McGill referred to it as "cosmic consciousness," inferring a connection to the cosmos, or universe. This creates an ethereal quality far removed from the limitations of a mere mind-brain connection. But it also explains some quirks of consciousness that may be related to *cosmic awareness*.

Cosmic consciousness may underlie some common phenomena which science has been unable to explain empirically. For instance, consider the inexplicable "gut feeling" that subsequently turns out to be true. Or you reminisce about someone you haven't seen in a long time, and she happens to phone you soon afterward. At the extreme are near-death experiences (NDEs), in which an individual pronounced dead miraculously revives and then gives a vivid account of what she experienced during her "death."

There is so much that remains unknown and, therefore, much to explore related to this thing we call "life." I am prepared to accept that consciousness is larger than the sum of brain cell activity and that human experience is more profound than what current science can justify via the five human senses. I am willing to entertain the notion of a sixth sense (or more!) and the new science of consciousness.

What is the possible nature of this sixth sense? Hypnosis expands the intuitive portion of your consciousness. But it exceeds the popular notion of extrasensory perception (ESP), allowing you to revisit past experiences (*recall*) with full emotional symphony (*abreaction*). *Abreaction* refers to sensations and emotions experienced during recall—in trance—that are a full and authentic representation of the original event. It is like reliving your life again in that slice of time. Yes, it can be painful, but it leads to the resolution of past hurts and allows past traumas to be *reframed*. In other words, with the aid of a skilled hypnotherapist, you can *rescript* an experience—applying an adult perspective to an event that occurred when you were a child, ascribing motivations to someone else's fears as opposed to making assumptions about personal inadequacies; or, in contrast, analyzing how your own habits of mind contributed to a failed relationship. The reframing process does not negate the original experiences but, rather, gets you *unstuck* so that those experiences stop holding you back from your current dreams and aspirations. All this occurs without the use of drugs or invasive equipment. The hypnotherapist simply guides you through the events and then helps you heal your hurts. Imagine traveling back in time to resolve an issue while sitting in a chair? Impossible? Find out.

Spectrum of consciousness

Figure 1 shows the spectrum of human consciousness as I imagine it. I have taken the liberty of extrapolating the EEG pattern described earlier to a continuum from wakeful, conscious awareness to comatose unconsciousness. The model is arbitrary, but it helps in visualizing how trance works.

Figure One. Neill's Spectrum of Human Consciousness

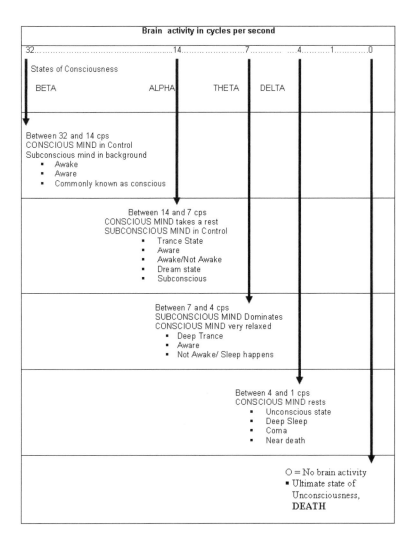

Imagine *consciousness* as the capacity to experience and process sensory information from within your environment. It's easy to presume this to be a dichotomous variable where *awake* = *conscious* and *asleep* = *unconscious*. But the context of a *continuum* of awareness suggests that you are *more* or *less* aware of sensory input at any given time. Responding to an alarm clock suggests that you are receptive to sensory input while asleep, and therefore conscious, though not very. So *asleep* ≠ *unconscious* unless the sleep is deep enough that you respond to no sensory stimuli at all (i.e., can't be awakened; unconscious). In other words, we receive sensory input and process information whether we are physically awake or not.

The *continuum of awareness* depicts *consciousness* mainly as a contrast between the *conscious* and *subconscious* minds. Taken to extremes, it goes from fully awake to comatose and even dead (the ultimate unconscious state), with wakefulness represented by a measure of brain activity in cycles per second (cps). However, that contrast means that at any point along the continuum, the interaction of the *conscious* and *subconscious* minds varies. At a higher cps, the conscious mind predominates, but the subconscious mind still has an influence on information processing and decision-making. At a lower cps, the subconscious mind predominates.

The relevance of that predominance becomes apparent when you understand that the *conscious* and *subconscious* minds are responsible for different types of information processing. The conscious mind is oriented toward *cognitive* processing. It deals mostly with objective facts and data. In contrast, the subconscious mind is oriented toward *affective* (social/relational) processing. It deals with subjective emotions and feelings. Therefore, your state of wakefulness determines to some extent whether you respond to sensory input logically or emotionally.

When awake, brain activity registers in the range of 14-32 cps (*beta state*). That means the conscious mind is largely in control, with the subconscious mind playing a smaller role. As you relax, the brain slows to 7-14 cps (*alpha state*); the subconscious mind takes over, allowing the conscious mind to rest a bit. This is the state at which hypnotic trance engages. You are awake and aware, inasmuch as you continue communicating with the hypnotherapist, but this state opens the subconscious for processing, accessing past events and receiving new suggestions. Deeper relaxation can slow brain activity to 4-7 cps (*theta state*) for deep trance. Because the subconscious mind is so much more open, and because the conscious mind is inhibited in a way that it can no longer interfere with rescripting, according to some hypnotherapists, deep trance work is often the most effective at resolving long-standing issues.

Slowing further than four cps puts the brain into a state of unconsciousness. The conscious mind takes a complete break. Consider it a very deep sleep. However, in circumstances of illness, drug use, or trauma, when the brain is unnaturally slowed toward zero, coma can set in. At this very low level of brain activity, the conscious mind is inactive, but there is evidence that the subconscious mind remains active. Even conventional doctors encourage loved ones to continue talking to patients who have lapsed into a comatose state. The patient cannot respond cognitively but is likely receptive to feelings and emotions expressed through the continued attempts to communicate with them. And of course, there are numerous stories of people who, upon awaking from a coma, relate clear memories of what they heard around them.

The *continuum of awareness* represents the capacity for experiencing sensory input whether you are aware, awake, or even unconscious. The proportional roles of the conscious mind and subconscious mind determine how you respond to that input. The relevance to hypnotherapy is that the subconscious mind is where experiences are reframed, which redirects the conscious mind to new patterns of thought and behavior, a path toward better health and happiness.

Trance is natural

Hypnotic consciousness is colloquially known as *trance*. Some hypnotherapists have tried to introduce terminology that is more accurate, and perhaps less sinister; yet *trance* remains the almost ubiquitous word used to describe the state of consciousness that characterizes hypnosis. Sometimes, people are concerned about the use of the word *altered* since it implies *changed*. Simply put, hypnosis is one of several levels of awareness. It is like changing gears in the car; different gears move the vehicle at different speeds, each giving you a different experience. But it is all within the natural capacity of that vehicle.

So there you have it. Hypnosis is natural. It is an *other* version of consciousness. You can invoke it and experience it if and when you wish. Because it is natural, hypnosis is safe. It feels pleasant, and there is nothing to fear because you have full charge of your own experience. You get to drive. Only, in a therapeutic setting, you also get a driving instructor.

Stop thinking

As described within the continuum of awareness, *trance* falls somewhere between *conscious* and *unconscious* awareness. While being conscious and cognitively aware is diametrically different from being unconscious, subconscious awareness splits the difference, exhibiting characteristics from both ends. So the hypnotic trance offers a focused dimension of its own.

When in the altered state of consciousness called *trance*, you experience a split sense of awareness that is neither fully conscious nor unconscious. You are acutely aware of being in a different state in which sounds, sights, smells, even texture, temperature, and emotions arising from the imagination are clear, vivid, and enhanced. This experience of being acutely aware and yet not truly conscious (as we more commonly experience it) is *trance awareness*. You are also aware of being in two places at the same time. You are present in the instant, remaining conscious of your physical reality while simultaneously experiencing an alternate reality in your mind's eye.

As you go into a trance state, cognitive portions of the brain (which typically invoke the five senses) take a temporary break. Some judgment and logic functions of the wakeful mind are suspended. Some people consider the conscious mind to be the work of the front brain while the subconscious mind resides in the hindbrain. In trance, the subconscious comes to the fore as your conscious mind relaxes. The geography of where the subconscious exists is not important here. Simply that it does exist is the important thing.

Everyday trance

Frequently in hypnosis you are directed to close your eyes. That's simply because it is a lot more relaxing to do so. But open-eye trance is possible as well and is much more common than you think.

The following are examples that show how you go into trance during day-to-day activities without knowing that you have, in essence, experienced *hypnosis*. Just because we don't call it that doesn't mean that it does not happen. Trance happens every day, more often than you think. It is natural and there is nothing to worry about. Perhaps you've had the following experience.

Road trance

> *You're driving late at night and a song comes on the radio that momentarily transports you back to your first school dance. You continue to drive, maintain awareness of other traffic, and arrive at your destination while at the same time reminiscing about an event that occurred 5-10-20 years ago. You hear the song echoing around the gym over public address speakers. You see yourself as an early teen. Perhaps you were dancing with your first love. You are aware of the clothes you wore and your hairstyle (and wonder, "What was I thinking?"). You hear shoes shuffling on the floor as everyone danced. You may even get a whiff of the gym or popcorn.*

Such recollection occurs in an altered state of consciousness called *road trance*. Driving is often repetitive and monotonous, which relaxes your cognitive mind. That allows your subconscious to take a trip into your past. While experiencing *road trance*, you are obviously not unconscious or asleep. Rather, you remain sufficiently aware of your surroundings to continue operating a motor vehicle while simultaneously experiencing a separate reality. When you emerge from the trance, it's usually a pleasant surprise to notice how quickly time has flown by. The caution, of course, is to not get so entranced by the fantasy, or daydream, that you become a hazard to yourself or others on the road.

Movie trance

Another common phenomenon is *movie trance*. Maybe you cry while watching a movie. Sitting in a theater with a date shouldn't normally produce feelings of sadness or grief. Yet you find yourself crying as the movie transports you to a unique time and place in which you empathize with the characters. You can logically rationalize that the characters are only actors playing parts, yet when they perform well, you feel the emotions they feel and suffer the pains they portray. This altered state of consciousness is the reason most people attend movies, plays, etc. You seek that empathetic response, whether viewing a drama, a comedy, or even an action/adventure. And if the quality of the screenplay or acting fails to produce that response, you consider it a poor production.

Book trance

A good book gets you so engrossed in the storyline and the characters that you lose all sense of time. You actually *feel* the emotions ascribed to the characters. You experience fear, excitement, love, joy, dread, anticipation, relief; a whole raft of emotions welling up from a book. You develop mental images of the characters and of the locations where the story is occurring. All from the comfort of your reading chair. From this perspective, Aladdin's magic carpet is a metaphor for a good story. Aladdin experienced numerous adventures in exotic locales without leaving his "magic carpet."

Advertisement trance

Everywhere you go—in the city, in the country, along highways, on the sides of vehicles, on the sides of barns, on clothing, restroom walls, trunks of trees—ads are everywhere. Advertisements are an everyday phenomenon that insidiously implants hypnotic suggestions. Varying degrees of hard to soft sell are used to establish brand awareness and manipulate consumers into making purchases. And though many of us are aware of the manipulation, we buy the products anyway.

The repetitive and ubiquitous nature of advertisement is a form of hypnotic conditioning that subtly causes you to buy things you don't need, and in some cases don't even want. Yes, it stimulates the economy, but it may not be good for **you**.

Most advertising causes you to imagine you will experience circumstances similar to what an ad portrays if you buy the product. Perfume advertising, for instance, is particularly seductive. The models in those ads are like no one you know in real life. The women have unusual beauty that turns heads and causes jaws to drop. You see them in the arms of equally singular men. And it's common to portray them in elegant clothing, attending a posh function, or riding in a flashy car (if not a sleek jet). The ad subtly suggests that wearing the advertised perfume is integral to the fantasy. Who wouldn't want a piece of that experience! So you go out and buy the perfume in an attempt to recreate the fantasy. (Even though it's likely you'll get no closer to that fantasy than sitting in your bedroom in a flannel robe, daydreaming!) Men are manipulated somewhat differently. Beer ads often portray men as caring only about sports and behaving irresponsibly. While it's the polar opposite to the female example, some men do indeed fantasize about such a lifestyle.

Marketers use the state of suggestibility within advertising trance to sell products. Of course, *hypnosis* is never mentioned. Marketers are clever and know not to spook their audience. Yet it is trance work all the same. When you get bored watching the same commercial repeated for the umpteenth time, take a look with new eyes. Try to figure out what type of person is being targeted and how they are being manipulated via advertisement trance.

Subconscious Notebook

It's evident that trance occurs naturally under a variety of circumstances. The unique thing about hypnotism is that it *purposely* induces an alternate reality. A hypnotic trance entices your conscious mind to relax while making the subconscious more available and, therefore, more receptive to suggestion. It is like opening up a notebook, a blank page ready to be written upon. You can remove an old page you don't like and write a new one, choosing how the story of your life is portrayed. Hypnosis is natural; accept it, embrace it, enjoy it.

CHAPTER FOUR

Applications for hypnosis

Hypnosis in action

Hypnosis is commonly used to evoke changes in personal behaviors. The range of applications is quite broad. For example, it can be used to deflect exam anxiety, to alter addictive behaviors, or to help you get out of a toxic relationship. Or hypnosis can be used to achieve personal goals; to become more proficient at performing specific tasks, such as in a sport; to become more effective within a profession; or perhaps even to become a more understanding parent. Practically anything you can put your mind to can be influenced by hypnosis.

There are three major applications for hypnosis: Stage Hypnotism, Self-Hypnotism (commonly known as self-hypnosis) and Hypnotherapy (or Hypno-healing, the use of hypnosis for healing). These are described below.

Magic show

Imagine sitting in a crowd watching a performer on stage who, in some magical way, is able to tell people to do things, and they obey without question. The behaviors generate laughter from the audience—as when one person jumps up and mimics Elvis dancing and singing. This is followed by another person, who shouts at the audience to stop laughing because the hypnotist has implanted a suggestion that he is now the sheriff and it's against the law to laugh!

Stage hypnotism is a dramatization of the subjects' willingness to accept suggestions. It is hypnosis-in-action that takes place within a brief period of time. Willing subjects (Note: Everyone in a performance is a volunteer) are put in trance, and suggestions are implanted that influence their behavior. Because the purpose of stage hypnotism is to entertain, the behaviors are generally designed to be funny to the audience. The hypnotist has to work fast and effectively to keep the show moving.

Stage hypnotism is performed to impress an audience. Therefore, the suggestions must evoke a very quick and dramatic change in each subject's behavior. The hypnotist must be very skilled and quick-witted to sustain the effect and adapt to each subject, most of whom have never experienced a hypnotic state before. If the stage presentation is successful, the audience is greatly impressed and satisfied, the subjects "wake up" relaxed, and everyone has enjoyed good fun.

In the ranks of professional stage hypnotists, it is unethical, not to mention bad form, to use hypnosis to make fun of someone. It's imperative that stage hypnotists respect both the audience and their volunteers. They are honor-bound to observe the ethic of never taking advantage of their subjects' goodwill and never degrading them in any way. One of modern history's greatest stage hypnotists, the late Ormond McGill, once said,

> Hypnotism must never be regarded as a toy that you play with to entertain yourself. The human mind is a delicate instrument, which must be handled with great care and respect. Remember, the hypnotist has a legal and moral obligation to approach the performance of hypnotism in a completely ethical manner, and appreciate that the most important person in his presentation is the subject and not himself.

McGill stressed that the human mind is the greatest wonder and mystery in life; and hypnotism, natural as it is, is also magic! *Hypnotism demonstrates the magic-of-the-mind.* And, that is why stage hypnotism is so engaging. It is simply a magical show.

Self-hypnotism

Self-hypnotism is what it sounds like—you serve as both your own hypnotist and subject. But like everyday trance, self-hypnosis covers a range of applications, some of which are very subtle and others that are quite specific. Although the term *self-hypnosis* refers technically to trance states induced by you on yourself, it also commonly refers to the process of self-hypnotism. This synonymous use is evident in the following.

If you're reading this book, it's likely you have other self-help books on your shelf. The books you select are not a random choice. Rather, you have selected books that you hope will lead you to a greater understanding of a problem you are facing. That problem could be as specific as credit card debt or as general as just being *stuck*. As you read, you reflect on how passages are relevant to your own life circumstance. Those thoughts lead you to preplan changes you could implement in your life to overcome behaviors or habits you know are preventing you from being the best you can be. As preplanning, you don't form a specific plan; there are no steps or a timeline. Instead, you simply think to yourself, "This is something I could do." That affirmation alone creates a positive sensation as you work your way through the book.

Yet you finish the book, place it on the shelf, perhaps recommend it to your friends as a good thing to read . . . and continue your life unchanged. Later, I will describe the roles of your conscious and subconscious minds in determining your behaviors. For now, you need only to understand that you have addressed a conscious desire by picking up a relevant book and reading it; your subconscious responds positively by allowing you to *dream* of how things could be better; but the conscious mind reasserts itself by reminding you of how things *are*; and that conscious filtering prevents the subconscious from accumulating sufficient momentum to change habitual behaviors. The end result is that the book has made you feel better, but nothing has changed.

The subconscious involvement makes this a subtle form of self-hypnosis. From that perspective, anything you do with a conscious motive toward changing specific behaviors is a form of self-hypnosis, from reading relevant books and magazine articles to attending classes and seminars. If your desire is strong, and you accumulate sufficient relevant information, this may lead to change. Unfortunately, most people are unable to overcome roadblocks set up by the conscious mind.

Another form of self-hypnosis with the potential to more directly access the subconscious is through meditation and prayer. This strategy mimics aspects of hypnotherapy by eliminating distractions—e.g., sitting or lying in a quiet place and really focusing on a specific intent. Though rarely expressed as such, that narrow focus is a trance. And as you might guess, the depth of that trance—and, therefore, the likelihood of it producing desired change—works better for some people than others.

Of course, there are other problems with these approaches to behavior change. Unless meditation is coupled with extensive knowledge gained from reading, or otherwise, and unless you have the ability to creatively apply that knowledge to your own life circumstances, you may not know what to focus on—i.e., what changes you should effect. You may also unwittingly be focusing on the wrong things—things that are unreasonable, impractical, or that simply substitute one undesirable behavior for another.

That is when it is helpful to talk to someone more knowledgeable than you. It's common for people to discuss their problems with family and friends. But this is unlikely to produce real solutions since they may share many of the same problems. In contrast, *talk therapy* is a legitimate treatment employed by psychotherapists, but hypnotherapists consider it ineffective due to its reliance on labeling as opposed to solving.

Let's say the preceding are forms of self-hypnosis that are popular but result in very limited outcomes; what does more formal self-hypnosis look like, and how does it work? If you think you understand a problem you're facing and are able to plan a practical resolution, self-hypnotism can be used to *rescript* old "programs" (i.e., to update ideas fixed in the subconscious).

Keep in mind, the intent is to create positive lifestyle changes and thus alleviate suffering. That requires very specific solutions. So it's helpful to consult someone who can help interpret the basis of a problem and suggest appropriate changes. Then you need to know how to induce a trance on yourself to sufficiently promote and support those changes in your subconscious.

Many people can learn to induce trance on their own in a few sessions with a well-trained expert. Those sessions may also explore the reasons for particular behaviors and suggest solutions. Reading a book is rarely sufficient to accomplish either goal well or effectively. Imagine using a pair of scissors to cut your own hair. It is much easier, and you usually get a much better result, if you have a professional stylist cut your hair instead. There are things you are better off not trying to do for yourself. As convenient as self-hypnotism sounds, there are limitations. There are some issues for which you may not be able to implement appropriate resolutions entirely on your own. In such cases, it's helpful to seek the assistance of a trained clinical hypnotherapist. Then, as with most skills, the only way to become competent is to practice, practice, practice.

The majority of my clients initially complain that they have tried many different means of getting unstuck. They've tried multiple diets or smoking-cessation programs. They've read all the self-help books and attended conferences. Friends, family, and church groups have provided assistance or a sympathetic ear. A fair number have even come to me after giving up on medication or psychotherapy. It is obvious they want change and have thought about it a lot.

In most cases, the conscious mind has prevented any real or lasting change. The advantage of hypnotherapy is that it directly accesses the subconscious. Once that initial contact is made, the client knows what the true hypnotic state feels like and can be trained to self-hypnotize for reinforcement.

From that perspective, self-hypnosis is a self-empowering means of extending the influence of hypnotherapy. You hypnotize yourself to reinforce suggestions originally implanted by the hypnotherapist. Though those suggestions are the result of a collaborative effort between you and your therapist, the emphasis of self-hypnosis is on *you*. Most suffering in this life is caused by the choices *you* make—how *you* live, how *you* relate to others, and how *you* think others view you. Many of the ideas that drive behavior are spawned from thought impulses originating in childhood that are still perceived through the emotions and mental framework of a child. As an adult, these old, fixed ideas persisting in the subconscious no longer work. As unlikely as it may sometimes seem, there are many things *you* can do to help yourself overcome suffering and remove those blocks to your personal effectiveness. A high level of self-efficacy (believing that you have the ability to help yourself) is then necessary for self-hypnosis to work for you.

Self-hypnotism, for the most part then, is used for self-improvement. Effective self-hypnosis is a process of putting yourself in trance and then making suggestions to your subconscious for desirable changes. How wonderful it is to rewrite the scripts that govern your life! You really can. In fact, the *only* person you can change is yourself. Does all this sound like magic? If magic achieves what appears to be impossible in ordinary terms, then self-hypnosis is magical.

Hypnotherapy

Hypnotherapy is delivered by a professional who is able to induce a deep trance in order to facilitate some desired healing. It takes specific skills, knowledge, wisdom, and intuition to be an effective hypnotherapist.

*Hypno*therapy takes place whenever hypnosis is engaged by a professional as a tool to help you resolve issues. The consultation typically begins with an in-depth interview to identify what it is you want to change. The interview process helps you make that desire specific, but it also identifies what you are willing to "give up" for that change. The hypnotherapist then induces a trance state, within which you are guided to reframe the problem and initiate change. A more detailed description of the process is presented later.

One of several myths about hypnotism, as a therapeutic tool, is that suggestions implanted during trance overcome your will to smoke or to eat certain foods, thereby resulting in smoking cessation or weight loss. In truth, the effectiveness of such therapy very much depends on your own willingness to change. Further, hypnotherapy, as opposed to mere hypnosis, seeks to resolve issues or patterns of thought that typically support negative behaviors. And because human behavior is the result of multiple life experiences, it often requires more than one session to resolve a complex issue. The wonder of hypnotherapy is that it is generally a very quick and effective solution for many behaviors.

In addition, most people experience a very pleasant sense of relaxation while in trance and upon their return to conscious awareness. This contributes to feeling a profound sense of well being. At the very least, you emerge from trance feeling good in every way. There are no unpleasant side effects to the process. To date, there has been no documented case of anyone harmed by the process.

Hypnotherapy vs. self-hypnosis

Which comes first, self-hypnosis or hypnotherapy? It's a chicken-and-egg question. Some highly motivated clients come to me already having performed self-hypnosis. Others are introduced to self-hypnosis during hypnotherapy. Likewise, some are better at it than others. If you come to me already knowing how to self-hypnotize, I can help by identifying specific ways to use it or by helping you reframe issues. In contrast, I give neophytes self-hypnosis homework to perform between sessions. Clients with a high level of skill at self-hypnosis call me once or twice a year for a "tune-up." Clients with less skill see me on a more regular basis, relying more on me to induce trance for them instead of doing it on their own.

The important thing to acknowledge is that hypnosis, far from being something completely out of your control, is unique within every individual. Therefore, it's not important whether you learn self-hypnosis on your own or through hypnotherapy. Rather, it's the responsibility of the hypnotherapist to take advantage of your skills and accommodate your preferences.

Choice and Consent

It is common for hypnotherapists to assert that "all hypnosis is self-hypnosis." That means no hypnosis can take place without your consent. It is imperative that you *choose* to be a subject. Whether you hypnotize yourself or let someone else do it for you is a separate choice.

That doesn't mean you're always aware of some subtler forms of hypnosis. You may not have been aware of the various trance states described earlier (road, movie, book, advertisement) until reading this book. Some, like movie and book trances, you purposely seek out. Others, like advertisement trance, you have had less choice over simply because you didn't know it existed. Yet while advertisements do exert some influence, it is unlikely they have *compelled* you to purchase something beyond your means or desires. Even if you acknowledge that ads have influenced some purchasing decisions in the past, you can now make a choice *not* to be influenced in that way—to become a consciously critical observer of how ads attempt to manipulate.

The same is true as you engage a trained hypnotist to work with. Contrary to the "evil eye" myth, you cannot be hypnotized against your will. Even after hypnosis has been induced, you can choose to continue or stop. At that point, however, the decision is governed by your innermost self, the self that resides in your subconscious. Its rules are more basic and less rule-bound than your conscious self. That's why you find yourself doing things that, consciously, you would find physically or socially impossible yet stop short of acts that, deep in your subconscious, are immoral or unethical. That makes all hypnosis self-hypnosis. It is unfortunate that too often we are unaware of having such choices. But now you know.

CHAPTER FIVE

Path to health and happiness

Health vs. Suffering

According to the Dalai Lama, the purpose of life is to seek happiness. Many people mistake pleasure for happiness. As a health educator, I say the first step to happiness is to have an optimal state of health. Good health is usually represented as freedom from illness. It also includes the ability to perform day-to-day functions without assistance or medication. But that's the easy part. An *optimal* state of health begins with a feeling of power to choose. The power to choose infers that you have options, that you perceive multiple possibilities and opportunities. This lends itself to a sense of hope and purpose.

I use the term *stuck* to describe most people seeking out hypnotherapy. It generally means they have lost their sense of hope and purpose and want to get it back. Until they get it back, they are *stuck*, unable to move forward with their lives. I characterize that inability to move forward as suffering; in other words, it's the opposite of health. Assuming you have a reasonable state of physical health, and you are breathing, *suffering* is the biggest hindrance to health and happiness. Like health, suffering also manifests in several different ways.

Investment in suffering

What is the difference between pain and suffering? Pain is a physiological response. Suffering is an emotional response. The greater the emotional energy you vest in pain, the more intense the suffering. For the most part, we are conditioned to believe that physical pain leads to suffering.

But the converse is also true. Emotional suffering has the potential to bring about and intensify pain. For example, investing energy in things that bother you actually makes them more bothersome.

> *Margaret complained of a stiff neck. Further probing revealed a dysfunctional marriage whereby she described her spouse as being "a pain in the neck."*
>
> *John had an ulcer. John was also terrified of his boss and complained of being "sick to the stomach" every time his boss asked to talk to him.*
>
> *Virginia, who complained of hemorrhoids, had an overbearing mother-in-law whom she described as being "a pain in the a—."*

Louise Hay, in her book, *You Can Heal Yourself,* charts how pain in different anatomical parts is related to suffering from life situations. For example, people with spinal problems often feel they receive little support from their loved ones. So there are multiple manifestations of this problem. Yet at base, suffering is perpetuated not by other people or by situations as much as by the energy you put into that suffering. The more you think or talk about suffering, the more you are aware of it. But neither can you try to ignore it. The energy continues to accumulate, eventually manifesting in illness and disease. And you wonder why you suffer!

Mental expectation

To be clear, I am not talking about "energy" as a metaphorical abstraction. Rather, I've learned that energy is real and tangible. In fact, energy work is common to many forms of alternative medicine (several of which I describe later). *Energy medicine* suggests that emotional suffering brings on physical pain. The explanation is that physical pain is a projection of one's conscious awareness of discomfort. In other words, you are consciously aware of something (injury, illness, or even a social situation) that you *know* is supposed to be painful, so pain becomes a psychic projection rather than a response to sensory input. The mental expectation of pain, therefore, intensifies the suffering.

Say I poke your finger with a pin; you probably respond by quickly withdrawing your hand and crying out, "Ouch." Did it really hurt? In such cases, you are not responding to an actual physical sensation of pain; rather, your mind *anticipates* it. The quick, evasive movement is a reflex action representing a protective response from deep within the subconscious. The prick of the pin is felt, the sensation is associated with pain that may result should the prick progress to a sting or a stab, and you move to reduce that likelihood. If you consciously allow me to prick that finger with the same amount of force, you can inhibit the reflex, and you'll not say ouch since you are not expecting pain.

Some reflexes are hardwired into the subconscious at birth. Many of these are designed for protection, such as eye blink and sensations of potential pain, as I've just described. Others are learned via conditioning.

For example, *close your eyes and imagine I am about to touch your cheek with a red-hot poker. Feel the heat as I move it closer and closer. Soon it will make contact. Now, imagine the most excruciating, burning pain.*

I know, that wasn't a very pleasant experience. Did you flinch as you imagined the poker getting closer? I mean both physically and psychically. You may have actually turned your head a bit at the prospect of even an imaginary poker touching your cheek. And as you formed a virtual sensation of searing pain and burning flesh, it's likely you simultaneously tried to reverse that thought, to remove it from your mind. In that way, your mind has accepted the pain as real.

Where did these sensations come from? It's likely at some point in your life you have touched a hot surface or had a small burn. Your mind draws on such memories to form mental images. In this case, the image was entirely fanciful, drawing on your memories but not a representation of any specific event. And yet, though it never happened, and is unlikely to ever happen, your experience was real.

Consider how much more impact real memories might have. What if someone in your past has poked you with something sharp, sufficient to cause real pain! What if you have been seriously burned in a fire, so you have a full appreciation for the sensations that would accompany a red-hot poker making contact with flesh? Such experiences create a mental expectation should anything similar arise in the future. In other words, once you've had that sensation, the memory of it shades all potentially similar experiences in the future. Others, who haven't had the same experiences as you, will find it difficult to understand your responses to such things. That's where it's important to acknowledge that your perception becomes your reality.

We often think of conditioning only in terms of repetitive stimulus and response (such as Pavlov's dogs salivating at the sound of a bell because that sound had previously, over a period of time, signaled the arrival of a food pellet). But conditioning can also occur via a single instance if the emotional response associated with it is strong enough (more on that later).

The problem with conditioned responses is that they are reflexive. Once established, every time a particular stimulus manifests, you will respond in the same way. Just as earlier, when you cried out ouch prior to any real pain, the person seeking hypnotherapy typically is responding to stimuli in uncontrollable ways. Reflecting afterward, they know their responses are undesirable, even illogical, but they feel powerless to change. That's when pain progresses into suffering.

The concept of perceptions becoming reality works the other way as well. Above, you were anticipating pain where none existed. What if you could create a sensation of no pain where pain is an objective reality? In other words, if you *believe* the red-hot poker cannot harm you, it will not burn.

The challenge is to change how you respond to conscious awareness. What if you could change the expectation of pain to an expectation of comfort? Such a shift vests energy in a physical sensation of comfort rather than pain. Because hypnotherapy is an effective tool for promoting just such a shift, that makes it effective for dealing with pain control. In effect, you can bring about anesthesia without chemicals. Don't believe it? I have stopped using local anesthetics when I see the dentist. I self-hypnotize myself to go to a pleasant place during dental procedures. During crown work, and even a root canal, I've had to ask the technician to stop inquiring about my (non-existent) pain so I could concentrate. I've yet to experience any pain. But the real benefit is that I've been able to immediately return to work or other engagements without having to wait for the effects of an anesthetic to dissipate.

Hypno-anaesthesia uses a hypnotic trance state to help you maintain focus on a comfortable feeling in your body, thereby circumventing any suffering from physical pain. After all, since suffering is a state of mind, controlling the state of mind distracts your awareness of physical pain; hence, no suffering.

> *Hypnosis has been successfully used in place of chemical anesthesia in some surgical procedures. In April 2006, Dr. John Butler (hypnotherapist) delivered hypno-anesthesia to a patient undergoing a hernia repair. The procedure was aired on live television in London, allowing the whole country to watch. Immediately after the operation, the patient stood up and gave a TV interview. Avoiding the use of chemical anesthesia helped the patient heal faster and bypassed the aftereffects of toxic substances in conventional chemical anesthesia.*

During certain religious rituals, Hindu fire walkers in India go into a trance and walk over a bed of burning coals unscathed. The trance is necessary in order to prevent doubts arising in the conscious mind.

Of course, fire walking is an extreme example, but it shows how far the mind can be conditioned to perceive an alternate reality (in essence, to ignore pain and limit injury).

By the time fire walkers approach the bed of coals, they have no doubts about their ability to successfully accomplish the task. Just as the mind can be conditioned to a mental expectation of pain, it can be conditioned to expect no pain. The firewalkers fully believe they will not be burned by the coals.

That's true for us all. Behavior is a function of *beliefs* ingrained in the subconscious over time. If those beliefs are positive, you will exert positive energy that results in the reduction of pain and suffering. Unfortunately, negative fundamental beliefs fuel perceptions and behaviors that produce suffering. And it's inexorable; as I noted earlier, investing energy in negative emotions—whether consciously (constantly thinking or talking about it) or unconsciously (sublimating your feelings)—always contributes to suffering. Fortunately, the Dalai Lama tells us, "Pain is part of life, but suffering is a choice." With some effort, and having made a conscious choice, you can redesign your perceptions and beliefs in ways that reduce suffering and, therefore, get you unstuck. A process of reframing your beliefs allows habitual responses to life's challenges to be rescripted, in turn changing your behaviors.

Choose not to choose is a choice

Hypnotherapy is a profoundly effective tool because it helps you *change* how you feel and how you perceive your circumstances. It empowers you to reframe even fundamental beliefs. Such changes lead to modifications in your *behavior*. The thesis underlying this book is that everyone has the capacity to create change and promote personal healing. Therefore, suffering is a choice, but change doesn't occur in a vacuum. If you choose to reduce some type of suffering in your life, it must be replaced with something. So not only must you choose to change, but you must choose to accept new behaviors to take the place of the old. Further, as I've noted earlier, the hypnotherapist can lead you in the right direction, but you must take a large share of the responsibility for implementing the changes you desire.

Hypnotherapy is a collaborative process. Generally, it's not a good idea to just read about hypnosis and try to apply it without some practical experience. Some basic skills are necessary. For instance, even though the bookstores are full of recipe books and people presumably purchase them in large numbers, is it reasonable to assume that anyone really learns to cook from reading a book? If you've never spent time in the kitchen learning some basic skills, the likelihood you can reproduce a recipe as described is quite slim.

> *Perhaps you have a friend like mine. Exposing a serious deficit in her domestic education, she called one evening to ask how one boils an egg. Not giving much serious thought to such a simple query, I told her to place the egg in a pot, turn the burner on high, and wait for it to boil. I received a frantic call ten minutes later complaining that the egg had exploded and attached bits of itself to every surface in the kitchen. This seemed inexplicable until it occurred to me to ask how much water she had put in the pot with the egg.*
>
> *Though it seemed to me too simple a step to mention, water is a critical ingredient for boiling an egg. And had I been there to demonstrate the correct technique for boiling an egg, she would likely have understood the process much better.*

The same is true for self-hypnosis. Reading about it is not the same as having an expert hypnotherapist guide you through it a few times. Rather, in the context of hypno-*therapy*, self-hypnosis is really homework. The hypnotherapist teaches you how to place yourself in trance and recommends what you are to reinforce while in that state. Then, as in any instructional setting, on subsequent visits you discuss how it went, and the hypnotherapist helps refine your technique. Just as in cooking there are necessary steps and discrete skills that must be learned and practiced. Self-hypnosis is not a substitute for hypnotherapy. It does, however, make hypnotherapy more enjoyable and effective.

Coping

Pain comes in many forms. Physical pain is palpable and even visible. Emotional pain is less tangible though no less painful. Suffering is an emotional expression of pain that inhibits the experience of joy and reduces the sense that one is living a purposeful life.

Suffering often manifests as feelings of hopelessness or rejection, even a sense of abandonment. It's a feeling of being unworthy, unlovable, and a failure. Suffering arises from feelings of guilt, anger, depression, and despair. It is tolerated because there seems to be no choice. Yet it creates a feeling of silent desperation screaming inside your head. Suffering is a pain so intense it cannot be soothed, a fire so hot it cannot be doused, an itch so persistent it cannot be scratched. Suffering is a feeling of emptiness, a sense of being alone, even in a crowd. Suffering is no fun at all.

On the other hand, suffering is no more than an emotional response. You probably know people who live with pain yet choose not to suffer. Just as you know of people who suffer intensely in response to minimal pain. For many, the suffering without pain is the more difficult to endure. When you cannot tolerate the suffering anymore, you are ready to change. Hypnotherapy can help.

Genesis of suffering

Suffering is an emotional experience spawned from fear. All life is energy. Energy is manifested in either love or fear. All behaviors are therefore derived from either fear or love. Fear is exhibited in the form of anger, anxiety, and depression. Anger is a bubble of fear burst open.

Let's say a colleague, Jack, appropriated your idea, presented it as his own to your boss, and got credit for it. You feel really angry inside but are afraid to confront Jack. He asks you to join him for lunch, and you snap at him. He has no idea why you are angry.

The fact is you are angry because you are afraid of losing a promotion to Jack. He appears to be the better candidate on the basis of the idea he stole from you. You are afraid that in the boss's eyes, you are not good enough for the promotion. You may not even have been aware of such concerns prior to this event. But now, the sensation of fear is strong, and it arose quickly, so it shows up as anger.

The challenge is to turn the fear energy into love, so the anger will dissipate. But that means you need to feel confident and good about who you are. You need to reinforce feelings of competence and self-esteem. Instead of remaining angry at Jack, approach and confront him assertively about his behavior. Say to him calmly, "Jack, you stole my idea and presented it as yours in the meeting. That's not right. I want you to go back in there and tell the boss the truth right now. If you don't, then I shall, but I first want to give you the benefit of taking responsibility yourself."

Having love for yourself, instead of being afraid you are not good enough, empowers you to tell Jack what he did was wrong without degrading him. Tell Jack what you want from him. Also tell him that if he is not able to take responsibility and rectify the problem, then you will. Loving yourself is very powerful. No energy needs to be wasted in anger arising from fear. Try applying this strategy in a situation you may be experiencing yourself, and you will see how anger need no longer be your behavior of choice—you can choose love instead of fear.

Many people are raised to believe that sadness and anger are bad emotions that should be suppressed. While you feel free to express joy, you feel uncomfortable crying or, worse, when others cry in front of you. But suppression of sadness or anger is no good. They are natural feelings, just like joy. According to Gil Boyne, anger is either exploded (you know what this means) or imploded (internalized). Fear that rises quickly and is based on a sense of guilt or unworthiness is expressed as anger. When that anger is expressed in violent ways (explosion), it can hurt you, other people, or both, leading to further pain and suffering. If you cannot adequately voice or act out anger, the logical alternative is for you to swallow it. And we've seen earlier that negative energy directed inward can lead to illness or disease (implosion).

A feeling is a feeling; it is meant to be experienced and expressed. But what's the appropriate way to express anger? If you don't know, you are not alone. Most people lack the skills to express our feelings in ways that support their sense of self-worth.

> *Shortly after the Columbine tragedy, I taught a class on anger expression. As homework, I asked a class of junior-level health majors at the university to write down one hundred and one expressions of anger. I suggested they imagine a situation in which they were really angry. The 101 statements, or acts, were to express how they felt.*
>
> *When they showed up for the next class, I instructed them first to take a red pen and circle all the statements that indicated inflicting violence on another person. Second, they were to take a blue pen and underline all the statements that indicated violence towards themselves. Third, they used a green pen to circle any statements that contained no violence towards themselves or others. The outcome was shocking (though I should perhaps not have been too surprised). There were many red circles and blue lines, and very few green circles. For one woman, ninety-seven of her 101 statements directed violence toward another person while the remaining four indicated hurting herself. It is a tragedy indeed.*

Whether you currently explode or implode the energy of anger, you can learn ways to express that energy in healthy ways so as not to hurt yourself or others. Anger is fear. Examine any instance in which you have felt angry. If you are honest enough and dig deep enough, you will discover that the anger arose from a fear of rejection, abandonment, or some form of criticism. It all eventually comes to rest on the fear of not being good enough or of not being lovable. And if left untreated or unexamined, it's the beginning of a vicious downward spiral of fear; taking you through feelings of self-loathing on into behaviors that are self-betraying. That's why it's so important to transmute fear into love. If fear is not transmuted, its energy proceeds on an insidious, detrimental path, causing you, and others you relate with, pain and suffering.

CHAPTER SIX

Energy of fear

Fundamental fears

According to Maslow's hierarchy of needs, human beings need food, shelter, love, and safety in order to achieve self-actualization. The first need is food. However, operating on a full stomach is just the beginning. You need love and a sense of security (shelter and acceptance). You also need to have a sense of purpose. If you become an adult and have not yet developed a sense of love—first for yourself, then for others—it is unlikely you will feel accepted and loved by others. That produces a sense of insecurity. If you do not feel accepted by others, you cannot feel safe in their company.

When you lack self-love, you are not able to develop a strong sense of purpose. The absence of fundamental love creates space in your energy field for fundamental fear. And fear is fear; whether it is fear of failure, fear of success, fear of rejection, fear of abandonment, or fear of simply not being good enough. Fear makes you feel worthless and hopeless. Fear manifests in anger, anxiety, depression, and, worst, despair.

Fear energy must be transmuted in order to experience transformation. Happiness and health come from peace of mind and absence of fear. When fear is changed to love, you feel hopeful and at peace and more ready to experience a feeling of safety and excitement. When your own cup feels full, you are freer to be generous and kind, possibly helping others to fill *their* cup. Love is the source of health and happiness. Love changes everything.

Degrees of fear

Anger not expressed in a peaceful way begins to accumulate in the body. If you get angry frequently, it begins to feel like you are walking on eggshells most of the time. And if you do not have the skills to express anger appropriately, it *will* recur. Frequent recurrence brings on a state of anxiety, causing you to feel tenuous and stressed.

Living in constant fear, feeling you are *not good enough*, eventually produces a state of *anxiety*. You begin to worry that at any time someone will have an opportunity to judge that you are not good enough. This makes you feel like a failure or loser, simply incapable, regardless of your actual abilities or achievements.

If this feeling of anxiety is present more days than not, you become frozen in fear most of the time. Thus, compounding fear in anxiety, *depression* occurs and suffering increases. At its worst, you become so governed by fear that you lose motivation to do *anything*, giving in to the temptation to stay in bed and hide under the blankets.

But that's not the only expression of depression. For others, the fear of not being good enough causes you to strive unceasingly for perfection. You get very busy doing "things," working long hours, talking all the time, afraid to stop and be alone. You become a perfectionist workaholic. Of course, you derive enjoyment from telling others how busy you are. It makes you feel important or accepted. But at the same time, you are not happy.

At either extreme, even depression takes time off. There are occasional days when you feel good about yourself—not many, but once in a while. Those are the days when you realize what you are missing out on in life.

It's important to note here that anxiety and depression are clinical psychological diagnoses. The current discussion relates to them simply as emotional states. As an emotional state, depression is not a persistent condition; some days are better than others. However, if there is no respite from depression; if it becomes an everyday experience; it leads to a feeling of hopelessness. When eventually even hope is absent, you fall into despair. Despair is the most intense and desperate form of human suffering. But it creeps up on you so gradually you may not realize it until you're there.

> *To help my students understand the progression of the fear continuum, I use the following exercise:*
>
> *"How many of you have been bitten by an elephant?" No hands go up.*
>
> *"How many have been bitten by a dog?" A few hands go up.*
>
> *"How many of you have been stung by a bee?" Several more hands go up.*
>
> *"How many of you have been stung by a mosquito?" All the hands go up.*
>
> *"What did I tell you—it's the little things that get you!"*
>
> *"When one mosquito bites you, you may or may not notice. When you get a couple more bites, you scratch the itch. When five or six mosquitoes bite all at once, you get irritated. When a whole swarm of mosquitoes bite you all at once, you are completely overwhelmed. Fear works the same way."*

While interviewing clients, I draw a chart (Figure 2) to explain how fear works in most people's lives. I then ask them to reflect on the level of fear in which they live. Most clients easily point out the level they are at. I give them a colored pen and ask them to mark that spot, and I date it. After a few sessions, we revisit the chart. Clients are happy to see that, after their energies have been transmuted from fear into love, they find themselves at a higher level from where they began. Often they are off the chart and happily declare they are not scared anymore.

Figure Two. Degrees of Fear

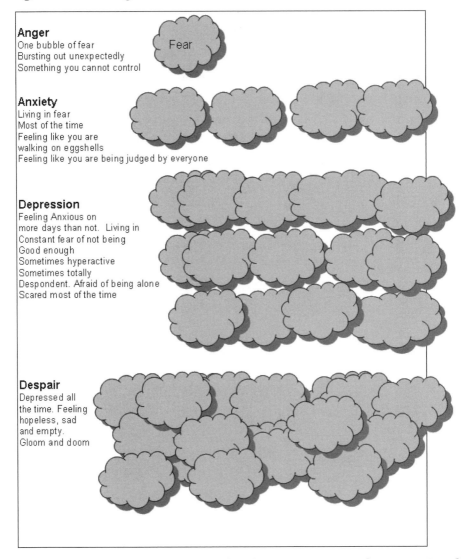

Anger
One bubble of fear
Bursting out unexpectedly
Something you cannot control

Fear

Anxiety
Living in fear
Most of the time
Feeling like you are
walking on eggshells
Feeling like you are being judged by everyone

Depression
Feeling Anxious on
more days than not. Living in
Constant fear of not being
Good enough
Sometimes hyperactive
Sometimes totally
Despondent. Afraid of being alone
Scared most of the time

Despair
Depressed all
the time. Feeling
hopeless, sad
and empty.
Gloom and doom

Most clients can mark a spot on this figure to express their emotional states at the time.

Hypnotherapy taps into your fears and changes them into love. As you become able to love, accept, and nurture yourself, you experience healing based on that transformation. It is a metamorphosis.

CHAPTER SEVEN

Choose to heal

Be exceptional

Health is indeed a choice. Louise Hay, in *You Can Heal Yourself*, clearly states that everyone has the power to choose to be healthy. As a health educator, I can attest that most morbidity is related to lifestyle choices. Returning to the wisdom of the Dalai Lama, "Pain is part of life but suffering is a choice." Your perspective of life situations determines your state of mind and, therefore, your state of suffering or enjoyment of life.

> *Imagine a cup containing 50 percent of its volume in water. Do you see the cup as being half empty or half full? Fact is, it's the same volume of water in the cup, regardless of your perception. I'd like you to consider a third option: it's the wrong size cup! I choose to have my cup run over every day. I choose to see life as a landscape of abundance. It is how you choose to see the world that determines how happy or healthy you are.*

There was a lady in her nineties whose husband had died, and none of her well-off children wanted to take her in. They decided to place her in a nursing home, where she would spend the remainder of her life. Despite the circumstances, she had lived a full and happy life with her husband, and she continued to feel blessed and abundant.

The day arrived for one of the children to drop her off at the nursing home. Tom, a young orderly, brought a wheelchair to take her to her room. He felt sad for her and decided to cheer her up by offering to wheel her around the facilities. She looked at the young man and cheerfully said, "Well, Tom, I am so happy to be here! I love my new home." Tom was puzzled. He noted she had not even seen her room. "How do you know that you will love it here?" She smiled and replied, "Tom, because I choose to be happy . . . it's my choice."

The power to choose is everyone's God-given gift. The power to choose is a mostly neglected and unused talent. Most people are blinded by fear to see the many options before them. They are so afraid to make choices that often they fail to make choices for themselves; they give over that power to others to choose for them. Who is better qualified to make choices for you than you? Are you afraid to take advantage of your own power? How sad that so many lack the courage to accept responsibility to choose!

Doctors are allowed to make extensive choices for patients, even to the extent of making a prognosis of death that may prove to be erroneous. The problem with this is that, assuming a patient accepts such a diagnosis—rather than asserting a choice to deny (or even resist) it—that acceptance may actually contribute to their imminent demise.

Granted, doctors are obligated to tell their patients the seriousness of a condition, but predicting death weeks or months into the future is unfair. It may be more prudent to admit having exhausted their knowledge and skills and recommend that you seek other avenues. Of course, this presumes that doctors may admit to their inability to cure.

I'd rather that doctors behave humanely than serve as messengers of death.

The courage to *choose* is a characteristic of exceptional patients who outlive their doctors' mortal expectations. Drs. Bernie Siegel and Carl Simonton coined the term *exceptional* to identify patients who choose to be the exception rather than the rule—to defy a grim prognosis and live.

So how you choose affects how you live. But where do you find the courage to choose? What makes you brave enough to exhibit that type of faith? That is when spirituality is put to the test.

I'm good enough!

Everyone has a unique threshold for pain and an individual tolerance for suffering. Unfortunately, fear of the unknown often outweighs suffering that has grown familiar. Perhaps one of humankind's greatest fears is *uncertainty*. Most people are reticent to take a chance or expose themselves to even a small risk simply because they fear the unknown.

This is commonly evident in the seemingly illogical behavior of abused children and battered spouses. Even though they know that staying with the abuser exposes them to continued pain and suffering, they cannot bring themselves to leave. Going to a shelter or a new home is unthinkable. They've developed a tolerance for the abuse that makes it bearable. And they cling to the hope that things will get better, that the abuser will change, become remorseful, and develop "loving" behaviors. Of course, it's all a rationalization for avoiding change, for the inability or refusal to make a choice that may lead to . . . happiness? This is more fearsome to them than you might imagine; because with the abuse, at least they know what to expect. How would someone who has never known a positive, affirming, loving relationship know how to respond when it becomes available?

Most people continue to suffer because they know of no alternative or because they have become comfortable in that state. And that's where many people resort to long-term medication (whether medically—or self-prescribed). Most acknowledge that the solace found in drugs and alcohol, et al., is only temporary, but while they think they're treating the disease, their tactics do little more than temporarily ease the symptoms.

Time to change

Suffering is cumulative. At some point, when you have amassed a critical level of suffering, it trips a threshold of tolerance, at which point you make a decision to change. Or: *when you can no longer stand the mosquito bites, it's time to do something about them.* When this readiness becomes evident, hypnotherapy is a very effective modality to guide the transformation from suffering to better health. In fact, it *only* works when you are ready to change. The necessary criteria for transformation are that you must be ready, willing, and desirous of change.

> *A woman phoned one day, saying, "I am so desperate to change. I need to stop smoking. I have tried everything and failed. I am so ready for you to help me. Please, help me. I know hypnotherapy works." Her conviction in the efficacy of hypnotherapy was surprising for someone who had never experienced it. And she did her best to convince me she was ready, willing, and desirous—right up until she asked about how much the hypnotherapy would cost. Then her tone changed dramatically, "Oh no, I cannot afford that! Thank you."*
>
> *What happened to willing, ready, and desirous? In my experience, when someone says they "cannot afford it," it's rarely based on a shortage of funds. Rather, they have other choices about how to spend that money, and maintaining good health or alleviation of suffering is not at the top of that list. Of course, it's not all just hedonism. A client like this likely feels she is not worth spending the money on. So the decision is based on poor self-worth or self-esteem.*

Whatever the reason, she made a choice indicating she was not really ready for change. On the other hand, I had a client who felt so compelled she emptied her savings account to pay for my services. She received the help she sought and got unstuck.

(I do not encourage anyone to go to such extremes, but it illustrates the different levels of commitment people exert to help themselves.)

Early in my practice, I offered my services to some clients for free, believing they lacked the resources to pay. I learned from that experience that anyone who was truly ready and committed could find a way to pay for my services. Those who, for whatever reason, did not or could not make an investment to promote change were less successful in the process.

It turns out waiving my fee was helpful neither to me nor to the client. Until you make the choice to change, until you take responsibility for that desire and are willing to give up something to make room for something else, and until you are ready to actually **do** something, a desire is nothing more than an idea. Desiring to change is not enough; you need to be fully committed to change.

There's the story of the chicken and the pig who passed a church as it was conducting its annual fund-raising breakfast. The chicken commented, "It takes quite a lot of commitment to put on an event like that." The pig, observing large platters of scrambled eggs and ham, noted, "You're only half right. It looks to me like some chickens were involved, but the pig was definitely committed."

Give up a blessing to receive a blessing

Nothing comes from nothing. You must give up something you have for something you want. Early on in my training in feng shui, I was reminded of the ancient Chinese tradition of lai see (blessing). The lai see is actually a red envelope containing something of value;

usually money, jewelry, or gold. Chinese people believe that one must always bear full responsibility for one's actions and pay for services and kindness that one receives. Red is the symbol of happiness. So whenever someone receives an act of kindness, there is a social obligation to return a lai see. The belief is based on simple physics: you cannot fill a cup that is already full.

I apply this in hypnotherapy. In order to experience change, you must be willing to give something up in exchange for receiving something. In other words, you cannot just add new behaviors, you have to be willing to give up an old behavior, or something associated with that behavior, to make room for the new behavior. That is the true nature of *change*.

My intake questionnaire contains two very important questions. One asks what you wish to change. The other asks what you are willing to give up in order to change. Life is a trade-off. Unless you invest in the process and take responsibility for your own change, hypnotherapy cannot effect any real change for you.

The lai see is not about the money; it's about *intentions*. Paying a fee to see the hypnotherapist is not the extent of your responsibility. Rather, you have a further responsibility to actually engage specific tasks that promote and solidify the desired change. I have clients who place their payment in a red envelope. They do so as an expression of their intent to follow through on what they have learned in their session with me.

White pill effect

I hope you are beginning to understand that what you get from hypnotherapy, and the potential applications of self-hypnosis, is really up to you. Anyone who seeks healing and change must be willing to do some *work*. As a healing process, you must take full responsibility for the work and, therefore, for the results. Half-hearted effort can only generate half-hearted results. It takes more than writing a check or reading a book (or lots of either) to generate healing. If you believe hypnotherapy works in a way that you don't have to do anything, you are mistaken. Hypnotherapy is only a path. It does not get you to your destination unless you place one foot in front of the other.

Writing a check is consistent with the allopathic model—the *white pill effect*. Write a check, receive treatment, and get cured. That approach allows you to avoid expending *yourself*, in terms of changing what it is that created and maintains your current state of discomfort. As a hypnotherapist, I can only facilitate your change; I cannot do it *for* you. I remember showing my children the potty and providing some basic instructions, but when it came time, it was up to them to *just do it*. Hypnotherapy can provide a certain amount of what, where, and how, but sooner rather than later, you have to execute and perpetuate change on your own.

CHAPTER EIGHT

Hypnotherapy is health care

Health care or medical care?

The scientific model of medicine is commonly referred to as *allopathic* medicine. Medical care as we currently know it works on what I call the *fix-it model*. Most people seek a doctor's assistance only when something is not working right. Usually, pain is the signal to seek treatment.

In allopathic medicine, the doctor holds most of the power. Patients acquiesce to them, ceding most of their own power in the patient-doctor interaction. That means patients make the doctor responsible for their health. Consider it an explicit contract in which the patient pays the doctor to diagnose the cause of pain and provide treatment (i.e., fix it). But there is also an implicit contract. Since payment transfers responsibility, patients perceive they have the right to *expect* that the doctor will determine a cause and remove the pain. But is that realistic?

Let's be honest, there is much in modern medicine that is not understood. It sits paradoxically on a pedestal of omnipotence while operating under severe limitations. Treatments and medications today are miraculous when compared to what was available even fifty years ago, but there is still much that remains unknown about illness and disease. And though modern, positivistic research has led to many of those advances, it has also narrowed doctors' choices to a range of "accepted" diagnoses and treatments. "Acceptability" is determined by research studies that establish a clear cause-and-effect as well as possible side effects. Anything that is not empirically measured or observed, or fails to achieve statistical significance, is generally outside the realm of accepted medical practice.

So what is a doctor to do when faced with symptoms for which there is no accepted diagnosis? The implicit contract makes an honest assessment (i.e., "I really don't know why this is happening.") impossible. So the doctor is compelled to give an opinion based on the proximity of those symptoms to something within his or her knowledge base. While that may provide short-term relief, it is not likely to effectively stop the illness or cure the disease. And until the root problem is addressed, the patient will continue to return with a series of new symptoms.

On the other hand, there are diagnosable diseases that have no known cure. Yet such prognoses should still not be interpreted as leaving *no hope for recovery*. Since no one can know exactly the path of an illness or when a patient will die, "time till death" is nothing but a probability, an estimate. Yet *nanosis* (a prediction of death) instills an instant sense of despair, which may be more disparaging than the illness itself. There is considerable anecdotal evidence of patients who die "on schedule," even when in a stage of biological remission or recovery.

> *On the other hand . . .*
>
> *Brad took his father to the doctor for a checkup. The doctor called him several days later.*
>
> *"Your father's lab results came back. I'm afraid I have bad news. He's got a serious illness and has only six months to live. I know you have a special relationship with your father. Would you like to break it to him, or have me do it?"*
>
> *Brad thought for a moment and mumbled back into the phone, "I'll do it."*

Five years later, the doctor ran into Brad and his father at the supermarket. As Brad's father ambled away toward the frozen food section, the doctor pulled Brad aside. "I'm so happy to see your father recovered. He seems to be in excellent health and good spirits." Then, pulling Brad a little closer, "By the way, how did you break the news to him five years ago?"

Brad got a sheepish look on the face, "I guess I sorta forgot to tell him."

The wonder is that while some diseases are quite intractable and resistant to accepted treatments, few are by themselves 100 percent fatal. While it may be true that a statistically significant number of people do indeed die from any given disease, there are still people who experience miraculous recoveries. It's unfortunate that many physicians share devastating diagnoses with their patients in a manner tantamount to a death sentence. But in a macabre way, it fulfills the implicit contract. One thing is certain—we all have to die. The doctor who predicts death, as in the case of a *terminal* illness, will be right sooner or later. No, it doesn't *fix* the problem; but it gets the doctor off the hook by making the argument that it's a problem no one can fix. Considering the alternatives that lie outside accepted medical practice, I consider the terminal diagnosis to be simply the result of an inability to consider new options.

Drs. Bernie Siegel, Carl Simonton, and Deepak Chopra would likely agree. They each describe "exceptional" patients who have defied dire prognoses. Such patients refuse to believe the negative and, through their own faith and those who support them, survive nanosis.

Giving physicians the power and responsibility for your health risks giving them the power to pronounce your death! Because patients expect doctors to "do something"—to prescribe pills or treatments—that is exactly what they do: they "treat the symptoms." The reality is that while a drug may alleviate pain, it doesn't really get at the cause of the problem. Further, buying into any serious prognosis means that even as physical pain is relieved, suffering continues.

Diabetes

With the discovery of insulin, it became possible for most diabetics to manage well and function almost normally. Few people actually die directly from diabetes anymore. Most diabetic issues can be managed by medication or surgery. Sounds good, right?

However, that means the need to find a cure for diabetes, while still important, is no longer urgent. In fact, the more efficiently doctors treat symptoms, the less there's a need to find a cure. So relatively few resources are directed at investigating a cure.

On the other hand, the industry of manufacturing and selling paraphernalia for diabetic patients has grown quite large. Economically speaking, finding a cure for diabetes would collapse an industry. Therefore, there is little economic or political capital to be gained from pursuing such an agenda.

The point is that medical care focuses on fixing what is broken, rather than preventing the break in the first place.

The Ambulance and the Fence

'Twas a dangerous cliff, as they freely confessed,
Though to walk near its crest was so pleasant;
But over its terrible edge there slipped
A duke and full many a peasant.
So the people said something would have to be done,
But their projects did not at all tally;
Some said, "Put a fence around the edge of the cliff,"
Some, "An ambulance down in the valley."

But the cry for the ambulance carried the day,
For it spread through the neighboring city;
A fence may be useful or not, it is true,
But each heart became brimful of pity

For those who slipped over that dangerous cliff;
And dwellers in highway and alley
Gave pounds and pence, not to put up a fence,
But an ambulance down in the valley.

"For the cliff is all right, if you're careful," they said,
"And, if folks even slip and are dropping,
It isn't the slipping that hurts them so much,
As the shock down below when they are stopping."
So day after day, as these mishaps occurred,
Quick forth would these rescuers sally
To pick up the victims who fell off the cliff,
With their ambulance down in the valley.

Then the old sage remarked: "It's a marvel to me
That people give far more attention
To repairing results than to stopping the cause,
When they'd much better aim at prevention.
Let us stop at its source all this mischief," cried he,
"Come, neighbors and friends, let us rally;
If the cliff we will fence we might almost dispense
With the ambulance down in the valley."

"Oh, he's a fanatic," the others rejoined,
"Dispense with the ambulance? Never!
He'd dispense with all charities, too, if he could;
No! No! We'll support them forever.
Aren't we picking up folks just as fast as they fall?
And shall this man dictate to us? Shall he?
Why should people of sense stop to put up a fence,
While the ambulance works in the valley?"

But a sensible few, who are practical too,
Will not bear with such nonsense much longer;

They believe that prevention is better than cure,
And their party will soon be the stronger.
Encourage them then, with your purse, voice, and pen,
And while other philanthropists dally,
They will scorn all pretense and put up a stout fence
On the cliff that hangs over the valley.

Better guide well the young than reclaim them when old,
For the voice of true wisdom is calling,
"To rescue the fallen is good, but 'tis best
To prevent other people from falling."
Better close up the source of temptation and crime
Than deliver from dungeon or galley;
Better put a strong fence round the top of the cliff
Than an ambulance in the valley.

—Joseph Malins (1890)

More than one hundred years after Malins wrote his poem, the philosophy of medicine has not changed much. Medical care is still more focused on *fixing the parts* that don't work (hence the *fix-it model*) rather than preventing problems in the first place.

One in three children in America is overweight. Children are now being diagnosed with diabetes Type II, a disease that used to only afflict overweight adults. So children are now being treated for what used to be considered an adult disease. Yet instead of spending resources on improving nutrition and encouraging them to be physically active, those resources go toward teaching school nurses how to deliver insulin to children. And finding a cure becomes even further removed.

America does not have a health care system. A health care system would help us care for ourselves. What we have is a medical care system for fixing the broken parts. While it is important to have a repair shop, should we not put some resources into maintenance?

More health care, please

Our behaviors determine a large part of our health, good or bad. Why is it so hard to change behaviors? The goal of health education is to provide the knowledge and skills to help people change their lifestyle. The goal is for them to adopt behaviors that help them become healthy and stay healthy. Health experts estimate that 50 percent of health status is determined by lifestyle, so teaching people to eat better, exercise more, drink responsibly, avoid drugs and tobacco, wear a helmet when riding a bicycle or motorcycle, drive safely, manage stress positively, and stay out of the sun leads to healthier lives.

Chronic diseases are among the top ten killers of Americans today. Because most are lifestyle-oriented, they are *preventable* for those who adopt healthy behaviors. Yet mortality and morbidity rise every year, so it's evident that knowledge does not change behavior. Further, attitude does not change behavior. In fact, even the threat of death does little to change behavior.

The leading causes of death in America are heart disease, stroke, cancer, diabetes, unintentional injuries, intentional injuries (suicides), lung diseases, and other chronic illnesses. Most recently added to the list is a source called iatrogenic diseases. *Iatrogenic* means unknown. That means more people who stay in hospitals or who see doctors are dying of unexplained causes. People are dying as a result of hospitals stays. Patients pick up deadly infections from staphylococcus bacteria. People suffer more or even die from staying in hospitals or as a consequence of misdiagnoses. Most of these ailments are related to lifestyle, including choosing the wrong caregivers, whether knowingly or unknowingly. Most are completely preventable, yet very little effort goes toward teaching and convincing people to take better care of their health.

Technological wonders have been invented to help doctors *diagnose* cancers, but there are still relatively few tools available to effectively cure cancer patients. When will we learn? Western scientists and physicians argue that technology has greatly advanced modern medicine. There are machines and computers that can see through muscle and bone. It's now possible to grow skin in a lab and graft it to a body. Surgery is performed on babies *in utero*. These are wonderful modern medical miracles, but they are all about *treatment* rather than *cure*.

In fact, it seems the more "advanced" medicine becomes, the further it is removed from helping patients heal themselves. Advancement seems valued by the human race, even though the result is a progressive inability to care for ourselves!

Please understand that I believe it is important to treat illness. And I'm grateful for technology that reduces suffering. However, I advocate for at least the same amount of energy to be exerted toward teaching *self*-help (my health educator soapbox).

Why does this approach seem to be ignored in traditional medical practice? Well, for one thing, pharmaceutical companies spend vast sums of money wooing doctors to use their drugs. For another, doctors are so overworked that writing prescriptions is considered the most efficient means of treatment, and of course, *time is money* in any business enterprise. It takes valuable time to perform extensive interviews that allow doctors to really connect with patients. The consequence of efficiency is that most patients find doctors uncaring and lacking in human connectedness. Yet few complain.

We are all too ready to get a pill from a doctor when sometimes chicken soup would do. Back in the old days, when you got a cold, mother tucked you in bed and brought you chicken soup. You took a nap and rested. Your body took some time to heal. You felt better. All you needed was some tender loving care, rest, and chicken soup. Till today, there is no cure for the common cold, but chicken soup still reigns as an effective treatment modality for all those who believe. Is this the health care you need? Sure tastes better than pills!

How long did your doctor spend with you on your last visit? How much were you able to tell her about what bothers you? Patients willingly let a person cut into their body who has spent less than ten minutes with them. Neither party seems to expect a person-to-person connection.

Yes, pharmacology is highly "advanced," but it's at the price of self-care. I disagree with the notion that we are a "healthier" society if that health is purely based on advancements in medical technology. After all, despite modern diagnostic tools and science-based treatments, we are no closer to eradicating illness and poor health. In fact, the overreliance on medical science to solve health problems may actually increase the incidence of poor health.

Think of patients who become dependent on medications and treatment. It's disconcerting that many current drugs (statin drugs for cholesterol reduction come to mind) amount to a lifetime prescription. Patients who end up becoming dependent on a drug for the rest of their life create an efficient source of income for drug companies. But of even greater concern, it diminishes the ability to care for yourself. The inconvenient truth is that the more "advanced" we've become, the less capable we are of exercising self-reliance.

In summary, the philosophy underlying allopathic medicine has not changed too much over time. It focuses on treating illness rather than promoting wellness. Bottom line, the business of diagnosis and treatment is more lucrative than the business of prevention and cure. The money stream ends if patients are actually cured. That's not to say that allopathic medicine is a negative force. Rather, while treatment of symptoms is indeed necessary, allopathic medicine would be an even greater benefit to society if it more compassionately addressed the *overall* health and wellbeing of all whom it serves.

True health care requires treating the patient, not just the disease, and doing so in such a way that you can take care of yourself as well. That means caring not only for your physical but also emotional and spiritual well-being to create a sustained sense of integrated wellness. I assert that modern medicine needs a little tender loving health care. Hypnotherapy helps you to take care of yourself. Hypnotherapy facilitates your healing. Hypnotherapy contributes to your health.

CHAPTER NINE

Alternative path to health

Alternative or complementary medicine?

Hypnotherapy alters the origin of problems in a way that allows patients to recover more *wholly*. Conventional medicine treats symptoms but rarely gets to the *cause*. Because the cause remains, other symptoms emerge to take the place of those that are successfully "treated." The cause is, in essence, a dependency manifested in the symptoms it creates. Conventional medicine too often trades dependencies, making a drug or other treatment a placeholder for the "disease." Since there is no real *cure*, you find yourself in a perpetual state of recovery, with no real hope for healing. Because hypnotherapy goes directly to the *cause* to promote healing, you not only "get better" but you bypass *recovering* to a state of being wholly *recovered*.

From that perspective, hypnotherapy does not fit the allopathic model in any way. It does not treat symptoms. It is not a "do for" modality, as in the traditional doctor-patient contract. Rather, it is a "do along with" therapy because the goal of the hypnotherapist is to help you help yourself. It expands your scope for *self*-care.

Complementary medicine consists of modalities that assist the modern medical doctor. Hypnotherapy is *more than* complementary. Rather, in many instances, it is an effective alternative. That would seem to be a bold statement, and it makes some people uncomfortable. But I am not suggesting that anyone stop seeing their primary care physician. There are many things they do well for which they are specifically trained. But there are also some things that hypnotherapy does better. In other words, hypnotherapy will never completely replace the services of medical doctors. But it has the potential to help many patients take care of themselves in ways that reduce their dependency on doctors.

You have a choice in determining how you maintain your state of health. There are many conditions for which hypnotherapy is a more effective mode of treatment than medical science. Clearly, I would not suggest you avoid seeing a doctor if you experience an acute injury (like a broken leg) or sudden illness. And if your day-to-day existence is dependent on pills and machines, it's unwise to drop them just to seek help through hypnotherapy.

Understanding the possibilities and limitations of both hypnotherapy and medical science will help you make decisions appropriate to your needs. Either way, you choose to take care of yourself or you don't. A broken leg will not heal well if you ignore the doctor's advice to keep weight off it and avoid further trauma. A broken spirit will not heal well if you ignore the hypnotherapist's advice to adopt new behaviors and practice new forms of communication.

I repeat, hypnotherapy requires that you take responsibility for your own healing. It is a viable healing option for all who dare. It makes you responsive to helping your body heal. It is simple, but you must engage wholeheartedly and trust the process. Halfhearted effort brings about minimal results.

Trust takes courage

The basis of hypnotherapy is trust. There must be strong trust between the therapist and the client. And both must implicitly trust in God or Spirit. That's the only way for any healing to take place.

I begin therapy by asking if clients believe in a higher power, something greater than themselves. They are usually surprised when I explain the question has little to do with their religion. Rather, I want to know if they have a sense of their own personal spirituality. In other words, do you *trust* the power of your God? Most people *believe* in God in one form or another, but *trusting* God is a whole other matter. And whether or not you trust says more about you than about God.

Jack was hiking up a mountain one day when he slipped on a rock and fell. As he was falling down the side of the mountain, he caught a branch of a tree. Looking down, it was a long fall. Looking up, it was an even longer climb. Jack had never been a religious man. In fact, he was agnostic. But looking at his options, he decided to take a chance on God.

"Hey, is there a God out there? If you are listening, God, I need your help. I will do anything for you if you can get me out of this. I will go to church, give to the poor, and stop swearing . . ."

As he tried to drum up more promises to sweeten the pot, he heard a voice, "Jack, I am here. Stop making promises you don't intend to keep."

"Hey, God, is that you? Is that really you? I promise I will do all these things, and I will do anything *if you can get me out of this!"*

"Anything?"

"Yes, anything!"

And God said, "Okay, Jack, I will help you." "Now, just let go of the branch."

Jack paused to think about it, then cried out, "Is there anyone else out there?"

Well, there is often a gap between our ability to believe and our willingness to trust. You see, trust is a choice. Within Eastern energy medicine, spiritual healing existed long before allopathic medicine or even science. Faith, trust, and the courage to act are the age-old ingredients for healing. Modern hypnotherapy contains these elements. Integrating them promotes *healing* for the whole person—mind, body, and spirit—in a way that medical treatment by itself cannot achieve.

Healing to be whole

Healing comes from the word *halen*, meaning "to be whole." Illness results when a part of you is not *whole*. However, fixing that part alone does not necessarily provide healing. As I noted earlier, pain leads to suffering and suffering can lead to pain. Suffering is an emotional state, and in that emotional state, you invest energy in suffering. *Well-being* refers to a state of health that is more affirmative than simply the "absence of illness." To heal in a way that restores wholeness, you must deal with both physical and emotional issues; you must redirect your energies from pain and suffering to healing. That is the basic philosophy underlying Eastern health practices.

In contrast, modern scientists treat the body as a machine. To them, illness is analogous to a machine malfunctioning. Figuring out what's causing the machine to fail suggests a way to fix it—i.e., mend or replace the broken part. Medical doctors act as biological mechanics, fixing parts within the human body as if each was static and unrelated to other parts. Of course, this practice is also deficient because it fails to address emotional and spiritual issues contributing to overall well-being.

CHAPTER TEN

A spiritual experience

Spiritual or religious?

Many clients ask about my religious beliefs. Some are simply curious. Others are concerned whether or not they should engage hypnotherapy, fearing it may be incongruent with a personal religious dogma. The therapeutic relationship is based on trust, so I gladly explain and hope it appeases their concerns.

First, I experienced a diversity of religions growing up in Malaysia. My family tradition is Buddhist. My grandmother spent the bulk of her time at the temple across the street and often took me along. My formal education began in a school founded by Anglican missionaries. From first through eleventh grades, I read the Bible as text. I learned it well enough that I represented my school in academic competitions on the Bible.

Malaysia's national religion is Islam. All radio and TV programming is preempted five times a day to broadcast Islamic prayers in Arabic. I grew up with many Hindu friends. I am now married to a lifelong Methodist and even sing in the Methodist church choir. Yet I have also spent most of my life as a scientist, a seemingly godless profession!

How do I mitigate all these traditions and beliefs? It is very simple: I believe in God, one God. By any name or description, God is the Universal Divine. Religion is man-made, spirituality is divine.

Spirituality is like the moonlight, *religion* is a box we somehow imagine we can use to capture a portion of that light. In other words, individual religions tend to place limits on spirituality. Meaning, even if you could catch a moonbeam in a box, you would only ever have a mere fraction of the moonlight. With as many boxes as you can imagine, we will never be able to capture all the moonlight. The implication is that God is much bigger than any religion. Spirituality simply refers to your belief in a higher power. Some people call this energy God, the Source, the One, or the Divine Universe. I believe that God is the Ultimate Energy, the life force that is ever-present in life in all its forms.

There are, of course, many different religions. In each, man-made dogmas tell that religion's adherents how to worship, what to believe in, and how to practice their belief. Too often, religious boundaries become a barrier to faith.

> *In seventh grade, I attended a Christian Scripture Union meeting. I had no understanding of what they taught, yet I was made to pray to accept their God and to become a Christian. I was very confused. One of my friends got very excited about her newfound religion, went home to her traditional Chinese parents, and destroyed the family's ancestral altar, greatly upsetting her parents and grandparents. My friend called her parents heathens and told them they would go to hell if they did not immediately become Christians. Even then, at fourteen, I knew there was something wrong with that scene. I saw how the attempts of the missionaries to "save" a soul had destroyed the core fabric of a family's cultural foundation.*
>
> *That could not be the intent of a loving God. It took me many years to get over the idea of an angry Christian God. Though I continued to read the Bible as text in school, the spiritual meanings escaped me.*

I believe that God is good. How can anything be good if it turns a child against her parents and her heritage? As an adult, I see that the missionaries failed to first seek to understand the culture they wanted to convert. In their zeal, they devalued and disrespected my friend and her entire heritage. Religion, in this instance, was presented as a box of dogmatic rules, rather than an all-encompassing divine love.

There is much more to discuss, but it would digress from the purpose of this book. Begging your indulgence, please entertain the idea that spirituality is much kinder and more accepting of differences than any religion can be. God is available to all who call. God is in every one of us, regardless of race, language, or gender. We are all equipped with our own little light derived from the big Light. Therefore, you have God in you, just as I have God in me. We can all be the same and uniquely different at the same time. Such is the wonder of life and the magnificence of God.

Hypnotherapy works better for you if you believe in God and better yet if religious dogma and fundamentalist beliefs do not place boundaries on your faith. It's important to have faith in a religion but also in the Creative Intelligence *within* that is derived from the *external* Universal Divinity.

Spirituality is faith that defies man-made boundaries. Healing comes from that faith and belief. If religious convictions create a fear that prohibits you from fully engaging in hypnotherapy, that therapy cannot produce healing for you. However, believing God wants you to be happy, healthy, and creative helps you gather the energy to engage the process completely to facilitate your healing. It takes courage and faith to be *spiritual*. Believing is easy. Acting on your beliefs is what enables hypnotherapy to promote healing for you. That requires trusting in your beliefs.

Everyone has the capacity to be spiritual; therefore, all are capable of self-healing. The real question is whether you have the courage to act on faith. Courage does not necessarily mean the absence of fear; it merely means you value something enough to choose it despite doubts or apprehensions. Do you trust yourself enough to act?

Hypnotherapy works if you are spiritual, believe you have the capacity to tap into the *divine* within you, and align with the Universal Divine Power. That Power enables you to transform from where you are to where you want to be. Hypnotherapy can help only if you are willing to act on your faith. It is that simple.

Gardener for your soul

The hypnotherapist, like the Eastern physician, is more a gardener than a mechanic. Instead of fixing broken parts, the hypnotherapist seeks to heal the person within and without. If life is like a garden, the gardener's role is to tend, weed, water, and nurture plants to help them grow. The gardener makes it possible for nature to take its course. The gardener prepares the soil, protects plants from pests and weeds, provides proper sunlight and water, and places plants in proper relationship with other plants so all have enough light, moisture, and space to grow. Under such conditions, the garden thrives.

Like the gardener, the hypnotherapist helps you rework unhealthy beliefs and reorientate behaviors, leading to a healthier lifestyle. Hypnotherapy returns you to times past to restore balance by removing ideas that don't work, replacing them with solutions that are more harmonious. It removes unfounded fears that have caused you to engage in maladaptive behaviors. From that perspective, the "hypnotherapist as gardener" removes weeds and replaces them with flowers.

You can affect your health by changing thought forms arising from your subconscious. How? The hypnotherapist guides you to rewrite stories within your subconscious. It creates a new garden on the same plot of land (you).

CHAPTER ELEVEN

Hypnotherapy Highlights

Alternative medicine

The thesaurus defines *medicine* as "pills, tablets, drug, prescription, and remedy." A *remedy* serves to "restore, or make it right." That makes hypnotherapy a kind of medicine because it helps restore peace, health, and happiness in your life. But contrary to pills, tablets, and drugs, it does so naturally, with no negative side effects. How powerful is that!

Hypnotherapy is an alternative remedy. Unlike most conventional medicine, it does not use mechanical equipment or chemicals. That means zero chance of chemical side effects. And it's physically noninvasive (no need to cut or poke).

Alternative is a more accurate descriptor than *complementary* because hypnotherapy acts alone to restore health and happiness rather than in conjunction with other treatment modalities. In fact, few therapeutic modalities are as effective in evoking behavior change in such a short time and with no side effects.

Natural medicine

What is most distinctive about hypnotherapy is that it is *natural*. It taps into your own natural abilities to heal. I often wonder why it has taken so long for Western culture to accept this. Hypnotherapy is a unique tool to help you feel better and heal. In contrast to allopathic medicine, hypnotherapy does not claim to cure anything, nor does it claim to treat any illness. Neither is it mental health treatment. And with the contrast I've described between spirituality and religion, it is certainly not *faith* healing. So what *is* it?

Hypnotherapy is primarily spiritual healing. That basis in *spirituality* aligns it with energy medicine and Eastern health care. Hypnotherapy promotes healing by guiding you to changes by which you can help yourself. Using neither drugs nor equipment, it empowers you to take charge of your life. It is a self-sustaining system of health care.

Spiritual healing

Hypnotherapy helps reconnect your individual divinity with the Universal Divine. That establishes a better sense of spiritual health. The result is an increased ability to evoke behavior change for disorders that might otherwise be characterized as emotional or mental illness. As a matter of fact, hypnotherapists do not make clinical diagnoses. Rather, they facilitate your desire for change without labeling your challenges. The most important thing is to get you unstuck and moving forward.

Hypnotherapy uncovers the reason(s) for emptiness in your soul. It locates the source of self-betraying behaviors. It retrieves missing pieces in order to help you feel *whole* again. Spiritual healing occurs when a feeling of being *holely* is transformed to feeling *wholely*. It is remedy; it is restoration. A feeling of *wholely-ness* emerges as your spirit is healed.

Belief in a higher power is what enables your spirit to be reclaimed. The healing is spiritual, not religious, which sometimes leads to confusion. People claiming to be "religious" usually assume they have a sense of a higher power. However, association with a fundamentalist religion makes "deeply religious" people leery to engage hypnotherapy, for reasons I've already described. I've found it possible to work with such clients by showing sensitivity to their fears.

I keep reminding myself, and the client, that hypnotherapy helps them find the diminished portion of their spirit, helping them to become radiant through the Divine (or by the grace of God). Reconnecting with your self helps reestablish faith in God (whatever your religion).

Hypnotherapy restores well-being in your whole person. It is true *heal*th care. Notice the word *heal* in the word *health*. Putting your spirit in order first sets you on the right path to taking care of your physical health and mental well-being.

Restorative power

Hypnotherapy empowers you to take charge of your own health and happiness.

Unlike conventional Western medicine—where the implied consent of paying a doctor relinquishes participation in your own health—hypnotherapy is a process that *requires* your full engagement, desire, action, trust, and responsibility. You have to take responsibility for your own healing, not just leave it up to the therapist.

Hypnotherapy enhances your spirituality and grounds your purpose in life. But . . . you have to want to heal. You have to be willing to change. And you have to be willing to act. Hypnotherapy is essentially a multifaceted, sacred contract between you and God, between you and the therapist, and between the therapist and her God. In choosing a hypnotherapist, it is helpful to know whether she performs her duties clinically or spiritually. It is best to find a hypnotherapist who can achieve *both*.

Effective and fast

The uniqueness of hypnotherapy is that, given the right conditions and a client who is ready and willing, healing is quick and effective. Conventional therapies can take years, yet hypnotherapy can restore well-being within five to ten sessions (10-20 hours). At the very least, significant change is evident in that time frame. Skeptics find that hard to believe, and most clients are shocked to see such fast results. But would you rather be surprised at how fast it works or disappointed that it did not take seven years! I have worked with clients who had been in mental health therapy for years with little change yet experienced a transformation within weeks of hypnotherapy. What is your choice?

The role of the hypnotherapist is to help you learn to take care of yourself. Too many modern treatment modalities include an element of dependency; hypnotherapy seeks to set you off on your own as soon as possible. How different is that! Would you rather be *in recovery* the rest of your life or *recovered* and moving on with your life?

To be *recovered*

Hypnotherapy helps you to be *recovered* as opposed to *in recovery*. Given the right conditions, and assuming you are desirous, willing, and able to act on a change, you can recover from being *stuck*. And I really mean *recovered*, not *in recovery*. Being *in recovery* means constantly waiting to fall off the wagon. In contrast, hypnotherapy teaches you to *drive* the wagon. It provides the keys and a road map. You are done, finished, empowered to carry on with life on your own.

CHAPTER TWELVE

Characteristics of hypnotherapy

The distinction in hypnotherapy lies in its unique approach to solving life's problems. Traditionally, we are taught to believe we can solve all problems by learning the answer to why. Hypnotherapy has a uniquely different perspective to human behaviors.

Why rather than *What* and *How*

The *Whys* behind behaviors you exhibit are not important in hypnotherapy. Knowing *why* doesn't automatically suggest *how* to remove *what* is causing the problem. To promote healing, you need to know **how** to separate from **what** ails you. Only then can you develop new ways to respond that are healthy and helpful. After all, if you've sought therapy, it generally means you're seeking a way out of suffering you can no longer tolerate. You want a solution, not merely the resolve to put up with something deemed intractable. In other words, you want healing.

Hypnotherapy uses hypnosis to help you achieve healing effectively. Since the hypnotherapist does not "diagnose," you receive no labels to hang your complaints on. On the contrary, you have to face your issues. But the hypnotherapist helps you by reframing old beliefs into new ones as the means to alleviate your suffering.

Hypnotherapy is effectively a goal and outcome oriented process in which the client and therapist collaborate. The goal is to relieve suffering or change negative behaviors. The hypnotherapist serves as your guide and facilitator, helping you figure out what does and does not work for you then using trance work to "rewrite the software" in a way that stimulates change. The outcome is an immediate change, in attitudes or behaviors, that removes blocks and reduces suffering.

> *Lani scheduled an appointment to ask for help with a weight problem. As the intake interview ensued, Lani disclosed that three years ago she had been a victim of rape by a stranger while she was walking through the park. Although legal justice had been served, and the rapist was now in prison, Lani's life continued to be a struggle. She had been in psychotherapy for the three years since but still could not get over the trauma of the event. Consequently, she had developed disordered eating habits, which had graduated to an eating disorder. (*Disordered eating *occurs when a person is obsessed with food most of her waking hours. That leads to eating excessively, in unusual amounts, or at inappropriate intervals. An* eating disorder *is a disease with more specific symptoms.)*
>
> *It turns out her marriage was in jeopardy, as was her sexuality. Knowing the* why *did not help her resolve the pain. The pain was emotional and spiritual. Lani went through about twelve hours of hypnotherapy, each session going into trance and regressing to the (*what*) piece of emotional trauma that had hurt her. In each session, I guided her to reclaim the spiritual part of herself that was left behind or stolen from her in the assault. With each session, she healed a little more. After each experience of retrieving her spirit, she felt more whole.*
>
> *Several weeks after ending her sessions with me, she cell-phoned to happily inform me she was at that moment walking in the park—and she felt safe! A few weeks of therapy was all she had*

needed to get her life moving forward again. Imagine, twelve hours of hypnotherapy compared to three years of psychological counseling.

Hypnotherapy facilitates changed behaviors, making you happier and healthier. Like a car, you have to drive it to move it. Sitting in the bus without a driver will get you nowhere. And letting someone else drive may cause you to arrive where you don't want to go.

I remember when I left high school; a friend wrote in my autograph book, "Anything the mind can conceive and believe it can achieve." Though she didn't know it, she was describing the magic of hypnosis. That inscription has given me the inspiration to be as successful as I can imagine. What good intentions my friend had for me! It was many years later that I began to understand how the human mind works in mysterious ways.

Most people seeking hypnotherapy are seeking to find ways to manage unpleasant situations or change unhealthy behaviors. Hypnotherapy helps alleviate suffering from physical pain, emotional trauma, and spiritual emptiness. It can help you lose weight, end abuse of alcohol or other chemicals, and terminate or modify relationships in which you have allowed yourself to be abused or disrespected. Hypnosis has also been used for persons in palliative care to eliminate the fear of dying and to help women have comfortable childbirth experiences.

Who can benefit?

Now that you know how hypnotherapy is different from other therapeutic modalities, you may wonder if it is right for you. Who can benefit from hypnotherapy?

Hypnotherapy has effectively helped thousands of individuals get over personal suffering from life situations. Here are some situations you may be experiencing where hypnotherapy can help you.

☐ If you know you are capable of doing *more* or *better*

☐ If you realize you are not happy in your current marriage or intimate relationship and you hope for something better

☐ If you are not happy in how you relate with family, friends, or colleagues and wish you could do better

☐ If you currently engage in unhealthy behaviors, abuse chemicals or yourself, and want to change

☐ If you sabotage your ability to succeed at tasks due to perfectionism or performance anxiety, whether in the bedroom or the boardroom

☐ If you are not as healthy as you would like to be

☐ If you have a chronic illness or think there may be options so you do not have to suffer as much as you do

The list goes on. No matter what you do, or what life situations you may be experiencing that make you unhealthy or unhappy, the feelings and behaviors above are manifestations of self-betrayal. When you don't act in your own best interest, you betray yourself. When you have no happiness, you suffer. So the choice is pain and suffering versus happiness and joy. I hear people say they can be happy without being healthy. I say you can be happier when you are healthy. And happiness is more lasting when you are also healthy.

Are you willing to entertain and act on *options* rather than remaining stuck with the *status quo*? Believe it or not, pain and suffering are optional. They are not inevitable. So you pop a few pills when you get stressed out or depressed. That's a convenient, short-term solution, but it doesn't solve anything. You stress over sport, academic, or professional performance, perseverating on the gap between where you are and where you want to be. That's just plain counterproductive. Hypnotherapy helps you remove the blocks that prevent you from getting where you want to go and being what you want to be. It helps you attain a sense of clarity about what you really want. It's like Windex, cleaning up the picture window of your life so you can see clearly who you really are and what you want.

Clarity of life and purpose help you enjoy this present life more. It rids you of fear, making it easier to experience peace and joy. Though the application of hypnosis is quite simple, its scope for solving problems is as extensive and expansive as your imagination. So back to the question, "Who can benefit from hypnotherapy?" The answer: anyone who is ready to change, willing to let go of the old to embrace the new, and ready to "Just do it."

Necessary dispositions

The mentality you bring to hypnotherapy is critically important. Your *desire to change* is the most critical element in the change process. No matter what a hypnotherapist does, hypnotherapy will not work if you don't deep down really want to change. Other dispositions necessary to experience "hypno-transformation" are: *willingness to focus* and *courage to take action*. You have to *want*, and you need to be *willing*.

Desire to change

Though often portrayed as such, hypnosis cannot create the desire to change. That desire must come from you. Clients tell me they desire to change, but when asked what they are willing to give up in order to experience change, they are reluctant. Unfortunately, there is no free lunch. A cup that is full can receive no more. Therefore, you must empty your cup before you can receive new blessings. This means you have to clarify what, specifically, you want to change and be clear about what you are willing to trade for it. You must be willing to give up the old to make room for the new. It is always a trade. You must know what part of your life and your identity is associated with any particular behavior and decide if you are willing to give it up and let it go in exchange for something more desirable. Nothing comes from nothing. The first law of physics is that "energy can neither be created nor destroyed." You cannot get rid of energy; you can only transmute it from fear into love.

The desire to change must come hand-in-hand with a willingness to let go of your old identity. A large part of who you are and what you do is connected to a personal *identity*. Unless you are willing to give up the old—die to your old self—it is not possible to create a new and healthier self. Your behavior defines your identity. If you have adopted a victim identity, you will have trained people around you to expect victim behaviors from you and to support that identity. Changing your behavior changes your identity. But that change also evokes discomfort in people who have become accustomed to your prior identity.

Hypnotherapy helps locate the energy you invest in fears and reinvest that energy to propel you from being stuck to being free and happy. So are you ready to give up the status quo? Becoming a nonsmoker could mean you have to find new social activities; you will not like being around your friends' smoking anymore. Are you ready for such a change? Can you give up your "smoker" identity?

Being overweight also carries many expectations from friends and family. A female who loses a large amount of excess weight may become a threat to girlfriends as they all go out clubbing. And family members can feel that their lifestyle is being criticized when you no longer share their eating habits.

Let's say you are committed, pay a fee, and schedule a hypnotherapy appointment. Does that mean you are really ready for change? While those are good indications, the rubber may still not make contact with the road. Your readiness for change is proportional to your willingness to let go of the old to make room for the new. Many clients say they are ready for change but discover during the intake interview that giving in to the change means they have to give up aspects of their lifestyle they had not considered. This is the time when someone discovers how willing they really are and makes a decision whether or not to proceed.

A fifty-year-old woman came to me for weight loss. We discovered during the intake interview that she had a fear of intimacy. My interpretation was that she had hidden behind an armor of adipose tissue all her life. While on one hand, she was lonely and longing for a mate, deep inside she was afraid of not being good enough if he did indeed show up.

Through an in-depth interview and some negotiation, I got her to accept her fear and to deal with it through hypnotherapy. As she worked to resolve her fear of not being good enough, she became increasingly aware that it was unnecessary to hide behind her fat. She began to eat more healthfully and started to engage in physical activity. This led to gradual, but natural, weight loss. As she gave up an identity of "I'm not good enough," the pounds rolled off.

Being fat provided protection for this woman, who feared intimacy. Making herself unattractive gave her a reason to avoid involvement with a man. Helping to rid her of the fear of not being good enough resulted in no more use for the armor of fat. Weight loss was a natural consequence of her behavior changes.

In another case, a sixty year-old man, who I'll call Mike, came to me for smoking cessation. His physician had told him to quit smoking or face possible premature death. We completed the first session, and I suggested a follow-up since he had smoked so long. At the next session, he reported he had stopped smoking but was struggling with the nonsmoker status. Since his hypnosis, cigarettes did not taste good anymore, but he found himself less happy than before he had quit smoking.

Further discussion revealed that as an older man who was single and wealthy, he enjoyed going to casinos to socialize. His current nonsmoker status meant he had to give up a very enjoyable social outlet. He decided he would rather risk his health and continue smoking than to give up his social life. He made a reasoned choice, and I returned him to his smoker status.

Willingness to focus

Assuming you establish the desire and willingness to give up an old identity for a new and happier you, you must then be willing to fully engage and focus on the desired outcome and the processes leading to it. Halfhearted efforts bring halfhearted results. The biggest challenge is to stay in the moment and not let your mind wander. That means being totally present and mindful of what you want to accomplish.

Staying "in the moment" requires you to focus on one idea at a time. You are *present*. You do not think about the past or the future. You attend only to what emerges at the moment. You have to be willing to simply mind your own business and deal with *only* the business at hand.

During hypnosis, you must suspend judgment. You cannot question whether or not you are in trance. You cannot filter responses through what the hypnotist might think of you (e.g., Am I doing this right? Did I say the right thing? I wonder how I am doing. So on and so forth.) Your mind may not ramble; it must remain still, stay put, and listen only to the hypnotherapist. If you can do that, it makes for a more effective trance.

During self-hypnosis, turn off the Blackberry and ignore the cell phone for a while. Keep in mind that you are learning a new skill, one that initially feels strange and ineffective. But self-hypnosis becomes easier to enter and more comfortable with practice. While there, it is again important to maintain focus on specific reinforcements.

Minding your own business means you must support your own changes and not get caught up in how friends and family respond to them. Acknowledge that change is a process. You will sometimes fall short of your goals. But if you maintain a strong focus on those goals and limit the inevitable distractions, you will experience the desired outcomes.

> Q: *How many therapists does it take to change a light bulb?*
> A: *Only one, but the light bulb has to really want to be changed.*

No more alibis

Wanting and willing to change are necessary preambles to change. Real change requires energy to activate. Many people have goals, and some people have plans. Guess who gets to the finish line first! Goals are merely ideas, wants, and desires. Goals sometimes are very strong. They motivate you to declare what you want and what you are willing to do to get it, but they are not the same as doing. And *doing* is where most people fall short. That's because they fall prey to alibis. The biggest alibi of all is "If." *If* only I had the resources, I could be successful. *If* only my spouse would change, we could have a happy marriage. *If* only I had not grown up in a poor family, I could be successful. *If* only I had been born with Tiger Woods's talent, I could play better golf. You get the gist. *If* is one of life's greatest hindrances. If you choose to find an excuse for not doing something, you can easily find a thousand more. Too often, more energy is spent making excuses and creating alibis than what it would take to simply get on with the task of doing.

People who plan, rather than simply set goals, show more willingness to take action in spite of their apprehensions or doubts. Yet planning alone is not good enough, either. A plan without a goal may get you to the wrong place.

> *Alice (of Alice in Wonderland) came to a crossroad in the woods and did not know which road to take. She asked the Cheshire Cat which road she should take. The Cat asked Alice where she wanted to go. Alice said she had no idea. So the Cat replied, "If you don't know where you want to go, it does not matter which road you take."*

Courage to take action

It is important to have a goal, plan for it, and take action. What does it take to actually *do*? What is stopping you from *doing*? It takes courage to change. Shakespeare's Julius Caesar notes that, "A coward dies a thousand times before his death." Courage is not the absence of fear. Courage is taking action in spite of fear. What does it take to step up and do something in spite of your fears? The reality is that success promotes just as much fear as the prospect of failure.

Change can only occur by choice. Choosing is the first step. Courage is when you love yourself enough to do the right thing despite uncertainties. Courage happens when you reinvest the energy of fears into loving yourself and trusting in God. Life is a matter of probabilities; only death is a certainty. Do you choose to live, or would you rather remain among the living dead?

> *Remember my friend who could not boil an egg? I suspect she had no real desire to learn how to boil an egg. Though I might have suggested putting water in the pot, she was too disinterested in the process to consider that the egg itself cannot "boil," which suggests she was unwilling to focus. And while one might argue she took action by placing the egg in a pot and turning on the burner, that took much less courage than enrolling in a cooking course.*

Trying is lying

Trying is a concept right up there with alibis or excuses. In *Star Wars*, Yoda admonishes Luke Skywalker, "No try, only do." Those simple words convey immutable truth. *Trying* leaves open an option of not doing. Any form of "I am trying" (I *will* try; I tried it, *but* . . . ; I'll *think* about it; etc.) is intended to absolve yourself from responsibility for failure (whether it's a failure to initiate action, a failure to follow through, or a failure to succeed). The assumption is that if you at least *try*, no one can fault you if you don't succeed. But in reality, it's all a lie. But it's not only a lie you tell me, it's a lie you're telling yourself. So trying is lying.

> *Suppose you ask me to come to a Tupperware party at your home on Tuesday night. The last thing I want to do is sit around, eat cookies, and buy plastic tubs. I already have too many (because I have attended too many Tupperware parties). But let's say you are my supervisor at work, and I don't want you to be angry with me. How do you think I will reply? You're right! "I'll try to come."*

And then what really happens? Right again! You won't see me at the party. It was an obvious lie because I made a "no" sound like a "yes."

But not all lies are as obvious, particularly when they're the lies you tell yourself. Nobody ever succeeds who *tries* to quit smoking, lose weight, quit swearing, or stop biting fingernails. How does anyone *try* to quit smoking? You either smoke or you don't! *Trying* allows the option of cheating—still smoking "a little bit" under the pretense that you've quit. What would you expect the outcome to be? Right again—you are still a smoker.

So, what's the alternative? Say to yourself, "I am a nonsmoker." (Think of it this way, "I am ~~trying to be~~ a nonsmoker.") *Do* it one day at a time. *Doing* is different from *trying*. Doing it often enough brings about the desired outcome—a new habit. So remember, trying is a form of lying. No more trying. If you are ready, you *do*. If you are not ready, you won't *do*, regardless of any treatment or intervention.

CHAPTER THIRTEEN

Hypnotherapy is transforming

M any people have the necessary dispositions and, therefore, the potential to create change on their own. The difficulty is to identify the nature of what is "blocking" them. In other words, they have the willingness and motivation but don't know *what* to change. The hypnotherapist helps identify blocks and makes suggestions for things to work on.

Discover your subconscious

Knowledge and memory are more complex than just "data in, data out." Rather, new knowledge is influenced by existing knowledge in such ways that everyone learns or remembers in unique ways. Further, everything in memory is charged with emotional energy. Taken together, memories crystallize over time into your own *truths*. Those truths subsequently form the maps from which your habits and destiny are charted.

If the idea of a personal truth seems too egocentric, think of an argument at a recent family gathering that began with two siblings' differing recall of a shared event in their childhood. If one of the siblings was you, you probably argued assertively for your own memory of the event while your sister argued just as strongly for hers. What's interesting is that neither of you was mistaken. In fact, others who were present at that same event probably contributed their own nuanced memories of it.

The nature of a habit is that you act (or react) in a predictable way, often unconsciously, and usually without knowing how or why the habit arose. But every habit started somewhere. I am suggesting that what you now experience as fixed ideas (habits of mind) have crystallized in the context of knowledge and emotions accompanying an event (or perhaps a series of events) you experienced as a child. It is as if those ideas are frozen in time. You can't imagine a different reality.

What's even more interesting is that, when you consciously recall such an event, you "feel" the same emotion you experienced at the time. Even though you can now assign an adult interpretation to the event, the memory of it still evokes the same emotion as when you were a child. And that memory leads you to perform behaviors consistent with what you may have expressed as a child. While it is obvious to an observer that such behavioral responses are no longer appropriate for you as an adult, they remain unabated until you find a way to reframe the event. Such reframing allows you to consider new options to replace old habits since you are no longer driven by the original emotion.

This raises a couple of important questions. (1) If the prior paragraph is true, I should be able to remember the event that initiated a bad habit. But I can't remember anything that led me to a particular habit. Why is that? (2) It sounds like memories last a lifetime. Even if I "reframe" the event, won't my memory of it still remain?

You are right—most people have no idea where their bad habits began. Part of the problem is that you have memories you are not aware of. The conscious mind is your *thinking* mind. It's where you retrieve knowledge and memories you are aware of. The subconscious mind, on the other hand, is your *feeling* mind. The emotions that accompany sensory information bypass your thinking mind and go directly to storage in the subconscious mind. Even though stored differently, emotions remain linked to the information with which they were received. But in every case, memories are "emotionally received." That means the emotion of an event is so much stronger than the cognitive aspects that the event can only be accessed via the subconscious mind. So you end up habitually responding to an *emotion* associated with an event to which you have no conscious access.

Memories do indeed last a lifetime, and as long as the emotion driving a habit remains fixed in the subconscious mind, that habit will continue—usually with a negative impact on your life. Hypnotherapy gives you a second chance at life by facilitating the process of reframing. It allows access to your subconscious such that you can replace fixed ideas (arising from childhood interpretations) with new interpretations based on adult maturity. In other words, memory of the event remains, but because hypnotherapy accesses that memory within the subconscious, emotions associated with the event are revised—meaning that the associated habit is no longer relevant to the emotional trigger.

Relationships, life situations, and health that are out of order cause pain and suffering for both you and those you interact with. The only way to reduce the pain is to change the behaviors that are not working for you. Hypnotherapy is useful in rewriting "the software" within your subconscious mind to eliminate harmful emotional triggers, subsequently replacing unhealthy behaviors with more healthful choices. Hypnotherapy supports true change while providing encouragement to expand courage, alleviate fears, and act on necessary solutions.

A formative practice

Since the days of Anton Mesmer (1734-1815), the manner in which hypnotism has been used to support healing has continuously evolved. But it has not been a smooth progression. Throughout history, the potential benefits of hypnotism have been overshadowed by the unscrupulous acts of charlatans. The misuse of hypnosis has, on multiple occasions, led it to be marginalized or even outlawed. However, with the advent of hypno*therapy* in recent decades, and the monitoring that now occurs via professional training and recertification, hypnosis is finally achieving greater acceptance as a professional modality.

Many modern hypnotherapists blazed a trail to make this recent acceptance a reality, including Dr. Milton Erikson, David Elman and Gil Boyne. Erikson discovered the power of the mind as a teen, and as a medical doctor researched many different ways to apply hypnosis toward healing. Elman lacked formal academic credentials but, nevertheless, as a self-trained hypnotherapist he delivered his own signature program to thousands of physicians and dentists. To me, however, the most daring of them has been Gil Boyne. Like Elman, Boyne is not a medical doctor. The contrast is that while Elman limited access to his training program to medical professionals, Boyne has taught anyone who shows a desire to heal others, regardless of background or education. Boyne is not grounded in the western medical tradition. Yet, he has talents and gifts that have allowed him to step out where others dared not. He is unconventionally educated, having studied with the best teachers in a variety of fields, with a single underlying goal—to develop hypnotherapy into a legitimate healing art. Throughout the 1940s and '50s he battled criticism from mental health professionals, jealous business leaders, and insecure colleagues. Yet, by the early 1960s, he had brought hypnotherapy to its current status, promoting it as a new frontier for healing, and almost single-handedly making it a legally recognized profession.

Gil Boyne originally conceived "hypnotherapy" as a rapid modality to help people transform their lives. His daring and creative rapid trance induction methods create transformation in the least possible amount of time. While most practitioners need ten to twenty minutes to induce hypnotic trance, Boyne produces it in seconds. Boyne defines hypnotherapy in his book, *Transforming Therapy*, as "a dramatically rapid intervention system, which strengthens and reshapes the client's feelings of competence and capability." By creating an instantaneous stage for change, Boyne's clients enjoy quick, effective, and successful outcomes.

But most important, Boyne weaves this magic quickly to get clients unstuck. He insists that hypnotherapy be *transforming*. Imagine being stuck in a behavior for most of your life and, within a few sessions, emerging with a new, optimistic perspective and positive behaviors that contradict former fears and suffering. There is no medical modality that offers anything similar to it. As Boyne says, "The true ministry of the hypnotherapist is to heal the self-induced blindness that has created a cloud of unknowing." In a manifestation of *I was blind, but now I see*, a metamorphosis occurs *within* the client, changing their entire demeanor. Further, the change is as permanent as desired. A "smoker" becomes a "nonsmoker" and never smokes again. A "nonstutterer" finds it easy to speak fluently. A once-insecure athlete sets new personal records. And a formerly abused and belittled spouse finds it possible to be assertive and pursue her own dreams.

All certified hypnotherapists are trained in the basics following one of several frameworks. In contrast to Boyne's transforming therapy, Milton Erikson's work led to what are known as the Eriksonian methods. Those methods have evolved into Neuro-Linguistic Programming (attributed primarily to Richard Bandler). Regardless of the framework underlying any hypnotherapist's training, each brings to the session a personal accumulation of wisdom and skill to deal with what emerges, to facilitate healing appropriate for each client. Part of the *art* of hypnotherapy is the creative use of hypnotism to help clients resolve their problems and get unstuck.

CHAPTER FOURTEEN

Hypnotherapist as professional

Goal for the hypnotherapist: To help clients alter their perceptions in a realistic way; assist them to believe in their own capacities to make choices to change self-limiting, delusional, and self-defeating patterns of thought.

—Gil Boyne

Bona fide profession

In 1975, Gil Boyne and John Kappas lobbied the United States Department of Labor to include "hypnotherapist" in the *Dictionary of Occupational Titles*. This was an important landmark for the profession. Their advocacy faced considerable resistance from the medical field. In the end, they were able to establish hypnotherapy as a safe and effective modality worthy of recognition and certification.

Inclusion in the *Dictionary of Occupational Titles* is important because it makes hypnotherapy a legal occupation. Hypnotism's association in the past with charlatans and exaggerated claims places a heavy burden on modern practitioners to hold its practice to the highest standards and conduct it with the most ethical and professional quality.

Hypnotherapy is a nonlicensed profession in America. The law only requires the licensing of an occupation when the unlicensed practice of that occupation proposes a threat to public health or safety. To date, no case of harm has been documented as having arisen from the use of hypnosis or the practice of hypnotherapy. Without a *need* for licensing, hypnotherapy remains a nonlicensed profession. However, as in any "profession," its practitioners master a body of specialized knowledge and skills to deliver a unique service. The key difference is that hypnotherapy doesn't require a college degree, as is common in more conventional professions.

Hypnotherapists are required to attain a criterion level of competency in skills and knowledge in order to practice. To maintain good standing, they must also subscribe to a professional code of ethics. Organizations such as the National Guild of Hypnotists, the American Society of Hypnosis, and the American Council for Hypnotist Examiners provide certification. Each regulates those they have certified according to their own code of ethics and accepted standards of practice.

Though the reputation and status of hypnotherapy has improved in recent decades, many academics and members of various mental health professions still decry hypnotherapy as an unacceptable profession. In fact, highly skilled hypnotherapists have helped an untold number of people, many despite having never attended college. In contrast, the exorbitant price of medical malpractice insurance is a constant reminder that there are mental health professionals who, despite extensive education and costly credentials, have caused unnecessary harm to patients.

Because hypnotherapists do not have the luxury of hiding behind a license, they typically uphold a higher ethical standard of practice through self-regulation. This is an alternative treatment—rarely covered by insurance—so they can hardly afford unhappy or dissatisfied clients. They have to work harder and better.

But . . .

Caveat emptor

It's always a good idea when choosing a hypnotherapist to first verify training, experience, and reputation. Then, the quality of your sessions depends on your comfort and trust in that person. You always have a choice. I recommend interviewing a hypnotherapist before engaging her services. Make sure you feel comfortable with her style and demeanor. See if she interacts with respectable and professional decorum. And if she tries to sell you anything unrelated to therapy, leave . . . quickly.

Who can be a hypnotherapist?

Certified hypnotherapists come from a diverse background, including physicians, health educators, psychologists, and psychiatrists. But there are also practitioners from a variety of healing arts and other mental health and health care professions. I have met hypnotherapists with former careers as airline pilots, engineers, air traffic controllers, and computer scientists.

Organizations such as ACHE set the standards for training and monitor the quality of training programs they approve. To retain certification, hypnotherapists engage in continuing education through their professional organization.

Of course, completing the required training is only the way to become *certified*. To be a true *hypnotherapist* requires extensive knowledge, skills, wisdom, and intuition. The effective hypnotherapist is true and sincere, having gone through her own "soul retrieval." That creates empathy for future clients' struggles and means she personally understands the sense of wholeness and well-being that can be achieved through hypnotherapy.

So an academic background is no guarantee of better therapy, but neither is desire alone. In the end, it is what the hypnotherapist *makes* of her accumulated knowledge and skills that makes the difference.

Though no one is perfect, the best hypnotherapists not only talk the talk but walk the walk.

> *Your talk talks*
> *Your walk talks*
> *But, your walk talks louder*
> *Than your talk talks*

CHAPTER FIFTEEN

Fundamentals of hypnotherapy

Hypnotism teaches you how foolish it is to accept any suggestion of failure, and gives you the ability to remain calm and relaxed, no matter how tense the situation may be.

—Gil Boyne

Making change happen

Hypnotherapy works via a very simple, but powerful, model of change that is based on seven fundamental ideas. Subscribing to these notions places change well within your grasp.

1. Behavior is a function of fixed ideas in your consciousness.
2. Ideas fixed in your mind by strong emotional energies remain stuck until they are *unglued*.
3. Fixed ideas are associated with the time period during which they were created (e.g., childhood) and produce responses according to how each idea was perceived at that age.
4. Fixed ideas created in childhood pose significant problems and suffering because the related responses are *not* appropriate for adults.

5. Hypnotherapy takes you back in time (*regression*) to the original event, accessing the emotion associated with the current response or habit.
6. The hypnotherapist helps you resolve emotional scars by leading you to understand the inappropriateness of current responses or habits.
7. The hypnotherapist helps you reframe the event and the emotion associated with it. This negotiates a revised perception that allows you to develop a new and appropriate response. That subsequently alleviates suffering.

Mary, aged seven, came home sick from school. Her mother made some chicken soup to comfort her. Mary loved chicken soup. She sat at the dining table and started to eat. Because she was already not feeling well, the food did not agree with her. A sudden wave of nausea welled up and, before she could get up and run to the bathroom, she vomited on the table.

At that instant, her father walked in the door. He had come home early, expecting important guests to arrive at their home soon. He saw the mess in the dining room and became very angry. He picked Mary up and spanked her. The more she cried, the angrier he became. The commotion stopped only when Mary's mother realized what was happening and came to her rescue, explaining to her husband that Mary was ill. By that time, Mary was inconsolable. Her mom cleaned her up and put her to bed.

Mary stopped eating soup after that incident. In fact, she began to experience a gag reflex every time she saw soup on a table. Over time it became even worse. She eventually developed a gag response at the mere smell of chicken soup.

Not being able to smell chicken soup, or eat soup of any type, posed a significant social hindrance to Mary as an adult. It was a problem she eventually realized the need to resolve. As an adult, she knew the ongoing fear of displeasing her father (related to a mess she made as a child) was irrational. But she wasn't able to overcome the sensation on her own.

Hypnotherapy helped eliminate the gag response. In trance, she was regressed to the event. While there, she was guided to reframe *it. ("Your father was acting on his own fear of appearing unworthy in front of important guests. It had nothing to do with you or the actual mess.") This changed the cycle by eliminating the irrational fear. After hypnotherapy, Mary was able to enjoy chicken soup for the first time in many years.*

Analysis based on Model of Change

1. Behavior is a function of fixed ideas in your consciousness.
   Mary's problem with eating soup originated with an incident from her childhood. Though the illness was inconsequential, her father's anger, and the disapproval it conveyed, made a deep impression that crystallized over time.

2. Ideas fixed in your mind by strong emotional energies remain stuck until they are *unglued.*
   The incident was charged with the emotion of her father's anger. It generated a fear in her of somehow not matching up to her father's expectations, of "not being good enough." Although she acknowledged the illogic of gagging at the smell of soup, she was unable to consciously overcome the subconscious reaction.

3. Fixed ideas are associated with the time period during which they were created (e.g., childhood) and produce responses according to how each idea was perceived at that age.
   Mary's emotions arose from an incomplete understanding of what generated her father's anger. She assumed it was the chicken soup, not the illness, that caused her to vomit. Further, her father's anger suggested she should have been able to control the impulse to vomit.

These are assumptions an adult would not make, but it's easy to see how a child might. The association with chicken soup stuck. Over time, it turned into a gagging response at the smell of any soup, but it was still based on emotions within the original event.

4. Fixed ideas that were created in childhood pose significant problems and suffering because the related responses are *not* appropriate for adults.

   Mary became a successful adult with no further need to fear her father's disapproval. Yet by that time, the gagging had become an engrained response. The real problem was that the gagging was not only irrational, but that it had made Mary socially awkward. This created a downward spiral in her self-esteem.

5. Hypnotherapy takes you back in time (*regression*) to the original event and the emotion associated with the response.

   Hypnotherapy regressed Mary back in time to the triggering incident. Experiencing the original emotion (abreaction; the fear she had experienced as a child) allowed her to make sense of her current behavior.

6. The hypnotherapist helps you resolve the emotional scar by leading you to understand the inappropriateness of the current response or habit.

   While in hypnosis, Mary was guided by the hypnotherapist to understand that the gag response was no longer appropriate for her. That doesn't mean the response was necessarily bad or wrong. In its original context, given her age and developmental maturity, it was an understandable response. But as an adult, it no longer makes sense to maintain the same emotional connection to soup.

7. The hypnotherapist helps you reframe the event, and the emotion associated with it. This negotiates a revised perception

that allows you to develop a new and appropriate response. That subsequently alleviates suffering.

The hypnotherapist guided Mary to reframe her father's anger as a symptom of his own fear. Seeing how her child's mind had misinterpreted the situation allowed her to conceive the incident in a new light. Once that was accomplished, it became easier for her to acknowledge that the gag response had been unnecessary all along. And with that understanding, she was ready to implement a more appropriate response.

She could also now see how her fear of not being good enough had contributed to the downward spiral in self-esteem. That understanding alleviated some suffering and prepared her to work on other issues as well.

It's important to note the client's active role throughout the process. The hypnotherapist does not "remove" a memory or independently "heal" the scar. Rather, the hypnotherapist facilitates the process of the client performing these actions herself. Of course, the hypnotherapist's knowledge and intuition are necessary in making a determination of what to do.

An emotionally fixed idea from childhood turned into suffering in Mary's adult life. The initial step toward resolving the problem behavior was when Mary realized that the *emotional response to her father's anger* was the source of her gagging response. Next, she had to accept that as an adult, she no longer had anything to fear from her father. But drawing those logical conclusions wasn't enough to overcome her irrational behavior. Consequently, the hypnotherapist helped reframe her perception and emotional response toward the original event. Now, with a new understanding of the event, and having changed the emotion associated with it, she was able to devise new and healthier behavior. Exhibition of that new behavior was a sign of imminent healing.

The role of the hypnotherapist was to help Mary go back in time to find the original scar. Once there, it took skilled guidance to help remove the scar and transform her perception and behavior. The transformation from fear of her father into love for herself was a profound change that brought about her healing. These are the mechanisms by which hypnotherapy works. Of course, the effectiveness of that therapy, and thus the persistence of the effected change, was dependent on 1) Mary's willingness and readiness, 2) trust in her hypnotherapist, and 3) the skill and wisdom of that hypnotherapist.

Changing long-held beliefs

> *Your thoughts become your words,*
> *Your words become your behavior,*
> *Your behavior becomes your habits,*
> *Your habits become your character and*
> *Your character determines your destiny.*
> —Source unknown

You *are* indeed what you think. As the saying goes, whether you *think* you can or you can't, you're right. Hypnotherapy is founded on the belief that all behavior is driven by ideas fixed emotionally in your subconscious. Ideas are encoded as *symbols*, not as literal or logical functions. In Mary's case, the smell of soup was a symbol of her father's anger and disapproval. The mind uses symbols as a means of generalizing recognizable events without fully or consciously attending to them. From that perspective, "jumping to conclusions" is a natural function of the subconscious mind designed to filter sensory input. In other words, you respond to most events unconsciously, without the benefit of mindful thought. This is an efficient process, designed to economize on mental resources. However, there are times when relying too heavily on symbols and not looking closely enough at facts or details is of questionable benefit (particularly to anyone who has been the subject of police profiling). Stereotyping has taken on a very negative connotation in recent decades, but for example, can you imagine the inefficiency of having to greet every new acquaintance as a potentially unique personality?

So the challenge is to maintain a balance between jumping to conclusions and overanalyzing every new acquaintance or event. Yet even if you know your mind is prone to jump to conclusions, it's not an easy habit to break by yourself. Assumptions driving those conclusions are based on emotional energy from prior experiences. The more rigidly it is fixed (either by repetition, or due to a single highly emotional event, as in Mary's case), the more deeply it becomes encoded in your subconscious mind. And that encoding is linked to your age-related emotional framework at the time of the event.

During infancy and early childhood, the child's brain is a relative *tabula rasa* (blank slate). As information accumulates, the subconscious mind directs the way the conscious mind responds to feelings and emotions. In other words, it performs the initial interpretation of descriptive information arriving in the brain via sensory input. Yet this process is not prescriptive because it does not process specific information—those are functions of the conscious mind. Neither does it evaluate or assess to determine logical connections or consequences. In this way, the subconscious mind is nondiscriminating. It simply receives data and sorts it for retention. So what goes in stays in until you go back through hypnosis and take it out!

At very young ages in particular, prior to the child's ability to sort information via logical relationships between pieces of data, information is highly associated with *emotion*. This leads to two potential consequences when subsequently accessing information encoded during early childhood. First, information provided by an authoritative source (what psychologist Lev Vygotsky called the "more knowledgeable other") will be stored as it was received. That's because the child cannot engage logical processes to discriminate between correct/incorrect, right/wrong, and good/bad. It simply accepts all information equally. Second, information is linked to emotions being expressed at the time it was received. Therefore, when accessing that information in the future, as a memory, the linked emotion emerges as well. The implication is that as a child grows, adults, caregivers, or even older peers in that child's environment "teach" the child, effectively writing the initial programming, or schemas, that direct responses to incoming information and sensory stimuli for much of the child's remaining lifetime.

> *Two five-year-olds are playing in the sandbox. John says to Mary, "Hey, Mary, in Mrs. Brown's house across the street there is a special room where all the walls are made of chocolate. You can peel off pieces of the wall and eat them." Terry considers this an interesting bit of information. That evening, she passes it along to her mother. Her mother is disappointed that Terry could be taken in by such a ruse and responds, "That can't be true. Nobody has walls made of chocolate." Then, fearing Mary might adopt the fantasy as truth, asserts more firmly, "That is not true. Mrs. Brown's house is just like anybody else's house. The walls are made of wood and paint and wallpaper." Terry is faced with now having to choose between believing either her friend or her mother. It's more likely she will trust her mother as the more authoritative figure. However, it may create some self-doubt. Contrasting memories have become written into the child's subconscious mind. Should someone in the future propose a notion that includes a house with chocolate walls, Mary will reject it based on her mother's opinion. Yet she may retain a sense of curiosity about it. Or she may have a lingering sense of embarrassment at having once been so gullible.*

Scripts, or schemas, created as a child remain with you even as an adult. Consider certain triggers that cause you to respond in a manner similar to when you were a child. Unless such scripts are replaced by new ones, you will continue to exhibit irrational (at least for grownups) behavior.

Upgrade the software

The important thing to note about hypnosis is that it is a natural, though altered, state of consciousness. You are not unconscious. During hypnosis, the logical, discriminating filter of the conscious mind is parked to one side, providing direct access to the subconscious mind. In this state of altered consciousness, your mind becomes gullible and suggestible. This makes you willing to accept new suggestions. Of course, it's usually better to remove a negative idea first and then replace it with a positive suggestion. It is always better to remove the old software in your computer before you install new ones. This limits potential conflicts between old and new.

Reboot the subconscious

The process works with even *deep schemas* (wrong ideas fixed in childhood by strong emotions). Think of it as loading an updated version of software. The new software overrides the prior version. But this analogy has further implications. When putting new software on the computer, it's usually necessary to shut it down and reboot. After a long session of *reprogramming*, it's not unusual for my clients to go home and have a very peaceful, profound, long sleep. They wake up feeling much better and very secure in their new behaviors. Much like the computer, we remove old ideas and upload new ideas, then take a rest and reboot.

Sleep is a natural state of rest. One theory for the necessity of sleep is that the brain uses that time to assimilate knowledge gained throughout the day. Without sleep, this assimilation would not occur; we would have no progressive learning. It seems that is what happens posthypnosis as well. You go home and sleep, giving the brain an opportunity to write new scripts, assimilating the suggestions.

Barbara drove two hours from Augusta to see me about an insomnia problem. As an out-of-town client, she planned to stay overnight at a nearby hotel. I scheduled a long session on Friday afternoon and a follow-up session at 9 a.m. the next morning. We finished our afternoon session around 6:30 p.m. Saturday morning I found myself waiting for her. She dashed in at about 9:05, apologetic but smiling. "I am so sorry to be late. I left yesterday and went to Wal-Mart to get some Epsom's salt for the bath you recommended. I was too tired to go to a restaurant, so I bought some food to eat in my room. Soon after my bath, I felt so relaxed I laid down to rest. The next thing I knew, it was nine o'clock! So I'm sorry for being late!"

"Barbara, you came to me to help you with what?" I asked.

"Insomnia." As the light of realization came over her face, she declared, "Wow! I guess I am cured!"

She told me later she had not had such a night of restful sleep in a very long time. We had worked hard Friday afternoon to resolve past issues and reprogram new behaviors. Barbara's mind rebooted overnight. I received a very nice thank you note two months later, telling me how well she had slept since that weekend.

It takes the brain time to process new ideas. As clients schedule a first appointment, I suggest allowing time through the remainder of the day to relax and do nothing. However, if that's not possible—let's say they must immediately return to their workday—I implant two posthypnotic suggestions. 1) "You feel excited and ready to complete the day's work." 2) "When the workday is done, you will go home and experience a very relaxing sleep." I round out the session with a final suggestion to call me in the morning and leave a message telling me how wonderful they feel. One thing is guaranteed—everyone leaves feeling well and relaxed, having experienced a very pleasant time in hypnosis.

CHAPTER SIXTEEN

Mechanics of hypnotherapy

Hypnotherapy step-by-step

A lthough delivery styles differ from therapist to therapist, key components underscore the hypnotherapy process.

Trust the hypnotherapist

Without trust, nothing can happen. Trust is enhanced by an office atmosphere that projects an ambience of comfort, safety, and professionalism—for example, framed credentials and professional attire often establish initial credibility. But rapport is also important. The therapist's vocal quality and eye contact, as well as other physical mannerisms, quickly determine whether or not you will establish a working relationship.

Integrate responsibility and response-ability

Unlike Western medicine, *hypno-healing* is a collaborative process. It begins by exploring your desires for change and clarifying your intentions. Most importantly, the intake interview includes a discussion of what you must do yourself for the process to work.

You must accept *responsibility* for your own healing. There are no pills to take, but you're likely to get homework. Commitment to that homework is critically important to the efficacy of the process.

Then you must believe in your ability to respond and accept change. That's not a given, even among people who seek out hypnotherapy. Some insist they cannot be hypnotized. They somehow expect that hypnotism is a contest of wills. They have a problem letting go of control because they imagine the therapist will take over their mind. They don't understand trance is simply a state of total focus and relaxation. So it is not a question of whether you *can* or *cannot* be hypnotized. Rather, *response-ability* is more a question of whether you are willing and able to focus and relax. You retain perfect control of your mind—all of it.

Spiritual work

The relationship between client, God, and therapist represents a *sacred contract*. All transformation happens by the grace of God. Little progress can be made if you do not believe there is a higher power to facilitate your change.

Inability to separate religion from God leads to a four-way contract (client, therapist, God, religion) that becomes untenable. That's not to diminish the importance of religion in your life, but things are less complicated if you are willing to place religious dogma aside while engaged in hypnotherapy.

My own clients sign a contract prior to therapy that ensures mutual agreement on these points:

I agree that . . .

o   *my health and happiness are results of how well I care for myself spiritually, emotionally, and intellectually, as well as physically.*

- *I will put my spiritual health first, before other dimensions of my life.*
- *The way I consciously or subconsciously feel, think, believe, or imagine ultimately determines how I choose, act towards, or relate to others.*
- *I am the only one who can take charge of my own life, and the only person I can change is me.*
- *blaming others, circumstances, or even myself does not contribute to my health or happiness.*
- *I am responsible for myself, my choices, and my actions.*
- *I can create and affect the happenings in my life every day.*
- *I will commit to being on time for my appointments and meet my financial obligations promptly.*
- *I am committed to participate wholeheartedly in the work I am undertaking.*

Energy work

It is important to establish a positive mindset toward the process as early as possible. Positive thinking is an initial step in creating a personal history of success.

You may be getting the impression by now that anyone who wants to change badly enough, and who thinks positive thoughts, will experience instantaneous transformation. That could possibly be true except for one thing—conscious thought. Don't forget, hypnotherapy works to change energy patterns and engrained emotions at the level of the subconscious mind. The conscious mind doesn't purposely interfere, but hypnosis gets around it in order to address the subconscious mind directly.

To further reduce distractions—to prevent conscious thoughts from intruding on the trance state—it is important that the therapy space be designed specifically to support trance. That is another reason for working in a harmonious and comfortable environment. My own therapy room is quiet, with colors and artwork on the walls that project a sense of calm.

I normally ask clients to empty their bladder just prior to trance work. It's easy to lose track of time while in trance, and I want to avoid an interruption by "the call of nature" during an important breakthrough. But this has a secondary purpose as well. Throughout the process of the intake interview and friendly chitchat, I tell success stories and express my own confidence in your response-ability. This contributes to a positive mental expectancy toward what you will experience in hypnosis. While directing you to the bathroom, I mention that upon your return, you should be ready for some very "profound work." This further reinforces that mental expectancy.

Suggestibility is willingness

To ensure successful trance work, it is common practice during early trance experiences to see if you are willing and able to follow instructions. I have known some clients to assertively claim they are ready and want to change, yet deep inside, they are not. There are others who struggle to focus. Still others are openly resistant, seeing hypnosis as a battle of wills or wanting to prove they cannot be hypnotized. Suggestibility tests ensure that neither you nor the therapist are engaged in a waste of time. The following is an example:

The Lemon Test

Close your eyes.
Imagine you have a slice of juicy lemon in your hand.
It is a very hot day, and the slice of lemon is cold.
You are very thirsty from the heat.
Place the lemon slice in your mouth.
Feel the sourness of the lemon juice explode in your mouth!

If reading this exercise made you salivate, you are suggestible.

Glued Hands Test

Place both palms together.
Clasp your fingers tightly.
On the count of three, imagine your hands are glued together. One,
Two, Three.
Try to pull your hands apart.
The more you try to pull your hands apart, the more they are stuck
together.

This test is more likely after you have been placed in trance. If your hands stayed glued together, you are likely suggestible enough to benefit from a therapeutic level of trance.

Relaxation routine

Sometimes it is called *fractional relaxation*. The following script relates a typical method of inducing trance. (Please do not use this to try to induce trance on your friends. Though not magical or overly complex, there are other steps involved in effectively hypnotizing someone.)

Make yourself comfortable in your chair. Place both your feet on the floor. Uncross your legs. Place both hands beside you. Focus on a spot in front of you. Take a deep breath, filling every cell in your lungs. Hold for one second then exhale slowly through your mouth. As you exhale, you begin to feel more relaxed. Take another deep breath, hold, exhale, and relax even more. On the third, inhale gently, close your eyes, and breathe normally. Pay attention only to the sound of my voice and only to my words.
Focus all your awareness on your left foot. Take a deep breath and let all the muscles and cells in your left foot relax. Now pay attention to your right foot. Breathe, and let all the muscles and cells in your

right foot relax. Notice a very pleasant feeling of relaxation gently move up your legs. Let both your legs relax. Now your hips relax. All your abdominal muscles relax. Take a deep breath now and feel your chest relax. Release all the tension in your neck muscles. Now feel loose and relaxed.

You can almost feel a warm, tingling sensation all over your body. Notice this pleasant relaxation now moving to your shoulders. Both your shoulders relax. Your arms relax. Now your wrists relax. You feel a tingling sensation in your hands and fingertips as both your hands relax. Now pay attention to the top of your head. Let your scalp relax. Feel a warm, pleasant sensation sweep across your forehead. As all the muscles in your forehead relax, your eyelids are totally relaxed and they shut completely. Now your face relaxes so your jaw is completely loose.

Now take a very deep breath. As you exhale, you feel this pleasant feeling more and more as you relax deeper and deeper.

The hypnotherapist will pause from time to time to check the depth of the trance. It's common to initially apply the "eye catalepsy" test.

"In a moment, I will count backwards from five to one. With each number going backwards, you feel this relaxation deeper and deeper. One: Deeper relax. Two. Three: Deeper and deeper relax. Four: You are so relaxed your eyelids are completely glued shut. You may try to open your eyes, but they are glued shut because this is such a pleasant feeling for you. When I get to the last number, you will go even deeper in relaxation. Ready, now. Five."

Depending on the purpose of the trance or the work to be done, relaxation is gradually deepened or compounded via any number of scenarios. For example:

- Counting back numbers: "Count backwards out loud. You will create a deeper feeling of relaxation as you continue to count."

- The Elevator: I suggest that going down floor-by-floor in an elevator will deepen the trance; then I count down the levels.
- Sacred Space: "Imagine a special place where you are happy."

The depth of trance is not always critical to the effectiveness of the therapy, though many practitioners prefer to put clients in deeper trance to promote healing. It is also common practice to give a posthypnotic suggestion at the end of the first trance session that, in future sessions, will cause the client to go into trance instantly upon a simple signal.

If you go into trance easily and repeatedly, you are probably ready to do some profound healing work. The first few times in trance are training or practice. Each successive episode of hypnosis becomes easier. Though healing work can be conducted in the first session, it can also take several sessions to get to the core of a problem before profound healing ensues.

Again, this is energy work, so it is not always predictable. The skilled hypnotherapist deals with what emerges during a given session, intuitively guiding the client to resolution, reframing, or healing as appropriate.

Promotion of healing

Once you are in a trance state, the hypnotherapist has a wide range of options to promote hypno-healing. Perhaps one of the most fascinating is *age regression*. This method takes your subconscious back to an initiating emotional event in your childhood that is currently causing a problem. As described earlier, you experience a state of *abreaction* while confronting individuals within the context of that event; only now, you are able to perceive it as an adult. A *split consciousness effect* allows your adult self to go back and rescue your child self. This occurs partly through *soul retrieval*, and partly through dealing with the situation as an adult. While "in the moment," you reframe the event, make adult choices, and adopt new opportunities for change.

Acceptance of the reframed event becomes a new truth, reducing fear by transmuting it into self-love, which subsequently transforms self-loathing behaviors into positive new behaviors that support your well-being.

Surprisingly, it may be initially difficult to accept self-love since most of us have been acculturated to believe that self-love is the equivalent of *selfishness*. But some reasoning and kind negotiation leads quickly to an understanding that acting in ways that support your own being does not require denigration of others.

Gretchen came to me for stress management. She was going through things at home that were depriving her of sleep. Gretchen was a retired schoolteacher. Her husband was also retired. Together they had good retirement income and no financial worries. Her husband wanted to travel with her and enjoy time together. She was too worried to go anywhere and felt she did not have the time.

They had three adult children, each with their own set of life's challenges. Gretchen also had an elderly uncle she cared for. She was a volunteer organist at her church, which was feeling more like an obligation. She sat on many community boards and committees. Though so stressed, she was afraid of turning anyone down or not jumping to serve others. The result was that she had no peace of mind, let alone time to travel with her husband. She felt overwhelmed and overcommitted but did not know how to stop.

In one of our sessions, she went back to an event which had turned out to be the last conversation with her father before he died. He said, "Gretchen, I want you to be a good girl from now on. Take care of your mother, your sister, and your friends." At the time, Gretchen was six years old. The mind of that six-year-old perceived her daddy to mean she had not been a good girl, and somehow that had something to do with losing him. Gretchen grew

*up to be a perfectionist and super caregiver, to the extent that she
neglected to care for herself.*

*Hypnotherapy helped Gretchen to perceive her father's death
with an adult maturity. As an adult, she understood that it had
nothing to do with her being a good girl, thus relieving her guilt.
But she also realized she did not have to please everyone to be a good
person. Further sessions helped her make choices that supported
her well-being. Sleep returned after two sessions. Gretchen began
to embrace self-love. After ten hours of hypnotherapy, she took off
on a long vacation with her husband, sleeping peacefully every
night. Self-love works.*

Reflection and reinforcement

You should receive some time before the trance is terminated to
reflect on how you have reframed events and changes you will make
toward self-nurturing behaviors. Use this time to ask questions and
clarify short-term goals.

Once you have experienced the power of hypnosis, you will probably
think of other issues you want to address. However, it is best to deal
with one issue at a time. Do not try to solve all your problems in one
session, but note issues to address in the future.

Just before termination of the trance, the hypnotherapist will likely
put in a suggestion to speed up the next trance induction. That is called
a conditioning process. She will also reinforce the new behaviors you
worked on through the session.

The end of the session reverses the beginning by gently "counting
you up." You "awaken" feeling rested and refreshed. You remember
all that has occurred—unless you don't want to—and feel excitement
about new prospects for personal health and well-being.

CHAPTER SEVENTEEN

Power of language and intentions

Start right now!

I don't know what caused you to read this book. Maybe you are overweight. Maybe you use or abuse nicotine or alcohol. Maybe you are experiencing difficulty in your personal relationships. You may be unhappy with your job or even your career. In some way, you are dissatisfied with the status quo and are looking for a means of changing your circumstances. It could even be that life feels pretty good, but you suspect something is still missing. Regardless, you know you can be more than the person you are, but you don't know how to make it happen.

I have suggested throughout this book that hypnotherapy is an effective strategy for overcoming these types of problems. It is a quick way to get you unstuck and move on with your life. And if you are open-minded enough to have reached this last chapter, hypnotherapy could serve you well.

The question is, what do you do now? I mean *right now*! It's unlikely that a hypnotherapist works just around the corner from you. And you may still not be totally convinced that it's the right solution for you. I don't want this book to simply join the other books on your self-help shelf. No, I do not want what you've read here to become a quaint idea. I want you to act on it . . . *right now*!

Personal energy work

If you recall, I have suggested that suffering results from mental expectations. Expectations begin in the subconscious as emotional associations, but they eventually emerge in the conscious mind as thoughts and words. Feelings of guilt, frustration, embarrassment, depression, etc. cause you to adopt language consistent with such thoughts. Your words express your truth, and that truth invests energy in suffering.

Let's contrast that with someone who has feelings of pride, competence, anticipation, happiness, etc. It works the same way. But words expressing *that* truth invest energy in joy.

That would seem to suggest that anyone having experienced a childhood of events charged with negative emotions is doomed to a lifetime of suffering. Not true. Energy is reversible. The process works in both directions. In other words, yes, a negative subconscious mental expectation expressed consciously in words contributes to a downward spiral of suffering, but the converse is also true. If you consciously adopt a positive manner of speaking, the energy within those words changes the mental expectation in a positive direction.

So the trick is to understand how the conscious and subconscious minds work, then exploit that knowledge to your advantage. How you choose to invest your energy has a tremendous impact on whether you can achieve wholeness of spirit. That's the essence of energy work, and you can do a good portion of it by yourself.

Genesis of mental expectations

The subconscious mind accepts and stores emotions and experiences just as they were received. It does not select or discriminate. And what goes in remains exactly as it was received until or unless it is accessed and actively changed. This subconscious input results in *scripts* that influence how you interact consciously with the world. Taken together, that means scripts retained in your subconscious are more than mere memories; they continuously influence how you interact with the world. Even old scripts, developed in childhood, continue to influence you as an adult. I have described earlier how hypnotherapy can be used to reprogram your subconscious—to create new scripts. Now I will describe how you can implement a similar process via a form of self-hypnosis.

Elephants, pain, and weight

Imagine your subconscious as a lifelong companion. You can't live without it, though it sometimes behaves in ways that distress you. It is prudent to learn how to relate to it directly and intimately. The subconscious mind receives only direct words. It does not recognize qualifiers or modifiers. Read the following slowly and do *exactly* as it says.

*Do **not** think of elephants.*

*Do **not** think of the magnificent, strong elephants of Thailand picking up logs with their trunks and dropping them into the river that transports them to a lumberyard.*

*Do **not** think about the royal elephants of India, that are dressed in silk and jewels to carry the raja and his wives in parades.*

*Do **not** think about pink elephants in the circus with the purple painted toes*

*And most important, do **not** think about Walt Disney's Dumbo, with his huge, droopy ears and tiny hat.*

What did you think about while reading that passage? Elephants, of course! Your subconscious ignored the qualifiers, all the *nots*. The only thing that registered was "elephants." In fact, further details caused you to think even more about elephants. Yes, your conscious mind was conflicted; "I know I'm not supposed to be thinking about elephants," but you got several mental images of elephants regardless. Now, try this.

> *Think of an animal that is small and furry.*
> *Think of an animal cuddles up next to you in a chair.*
> *Think of how that animal laps up water from a bowl.*
> *Think of how that animal playfully romps with its littermates.*

Were you still thinking about elephants? Okay, you may have briefly considered how different this animal was from elephants in the prior exercise, but the image of a different animal predominated. And that's the point.

If you want to stop certain thoughts or habits, you cannot just tell yourself what *not* to do. The subconscious does not allow such things to be negated or ignored. The sad paradox is that you cannot think or talk about a negative trait without unintentionally reinforcing it in the subconscious.

Instead, you need to substitute a more favorable thought or habit. For example, if you want to eliminate the sensation of physical pain, do not refer to "pain" in any form. Substitute, "I will feel no pain," with, "I am going to a place in my mind where all I feel is comfort and joy." Only the naive hypnotist says, "You will feel no pain." That statement draws the attention of the subconscious mind to "pain," producing the exact opposite of the intended effect. Skilled hypnotists are more likely to suggest, "I'm going to press this needle into your finger. As I do so, you will feel a slight pressure. Then your finger will feel as light as a feather."

Let's apply the same concept to weight loss. The naïve hypnotherapist suggests that a client, "will stop eating pie and cake." This sounds like an affirmative statement, but the subconscious doesn't register "stop." That is why diet programs fail. They focus on restrictions rather than alternatives.

However, the alternatives also need to be well-considered. I can suggest, "Pie and cake will begin to taste increasingly salty after three bites. By the time you've eaten seven bites, pie and cake will taste like pure salt." The salt taste is certainly aversive, but it makes the client no more likely to seek out healthier alternatives.

I tried this aversion technique once early in my hypnotherapy practice. The client returned with mixed feelings the next week.

"It's amazing how well the hypnotic suggestions worked. I was at a party, and the host offered me a piece of cake. It was absolutely wonderful. It's the type of cake I would usually wolf down and ask for another piece. But this time, as I began the fourth bite, I could taste the salt. I thought there was something wrong with the cake until I realized it was related to my hypnotherapy session last week. The next bite was even saltier. And I tried another but had to spit it out because it tasted so salty."

"So you're happy with what we did last week?"

"Well . . . not exactly. Can we add cookies to the suggestion this week?"

"You didn't mention cookies last week, or I could have included them then."

"They weren't a problem last week. And I don't normally even care for them. But eliminating pie and cake seems to have produced a craving for cookies."

The hypnotic suggestion had referred specifically to pie and cake. When those two items became unpalatable, her preference switched to cookies. Realizing my misassumption, I complied with her request to add cookies but went on to make a further suggestion.

*"When you leave my office today, you will stop along the way home
and buy a bottle of water. You will discover that you really like the
taste of that water. In fact, you like water so much that it becomes
your favorite beverage."*

Water did become a favorite beverage that gradually replaced sodas;
a further suggestion ended her desire for drinking sodas. Healthier
foods subsequently replaced pie, cake, and cookies in her "diet." But
after that initial revelation, the only thing I eliminated was the word
"diet." She lost weight not because she was dieting—a concept that
conveys restrictions and reinforces a negative connotation of *weight* in
the subconscious—but because she began to eat more nutritious foods
and engage in more physical activity. The emphasis was on what she
could complete in an affirmative way, as opposed to negations.

Power of words

Again, you cannot think or talk about a negative trait without
unintentionally reinforcing it in the subconscious. Perhaps more
insidious is that people introduce negativity unintentionally, and
largely counterproductively. Teachers tell students, "If you don't do
your homework, you will fail," "If I were you, I wouldn't do that," or
"Don't you even think about turning in an incomplete assignment!"
What do students do? They neglect their homework, think up things
the teacher wouldn't do, and turn in incomplete work.

Parents, who learned from teachers, frame their advice the same
way. "Don't play with fire" and "Stop talking back at me." And they
talk to each other the same way. "Don't cheat on me, or else." Filtered
through the subconscious, it's a pattern that invites the very thing you
want to avoid.

That doesn't mean everyone responds to the invitation. What
the admonitions do produce, however, are undesirable feelings. The
subconscious internalizes the negative emotions accompanying the
admonitions. Any "don't" statement presumes that the hearer is

likely to "do." Most "don't" statements, therefore, convey negative assumptions—negative energy.

~~But, don't despair~~ . . . (oops) But be of good cheer: if you are grounded, and if you have accumulated a wellspring of positive energy, you will either deflect negative energy within such admonitions or convert it into even more positive energy. In other words, energies you put into the way you think create your reality, not the other way around. It's much better to feel good about yourself than to rely on other people feeling good about you. After all, too many of the people you rely on to fill your cup are low on energy themselves. But if you maintain your positive energy, it draws others to you who also have positive energy. *Like* attracts *like*. Therefore, *fear* begets *fear*, and *happiness* attracts *happiness*. The rich get richer. Losers hang out with losers. If you think you can, or if you think you can't, you are right! Bottom line—you set the frequency and send out signals, and the Universe responds.

Cup half empty or half full?

Your perceptions become your truths. And your intentions become your destiny. Understanding this goes a long way toward improving your lot in life, but only if you're willing to examine those perceptions and intentions.

Did you know you can choose to think positively, to focus on the beneficial side of Life? If you see the cup as half empty, you will always feel incomplete. But you can also choose to see the cup as half full, feeling grateful for what you have. I suggest a third choice. It's the wrong cup! I choose to have a different cup altogether. I believe I own my feelings, and if I choose my own cup, I can choose to have my cup run over every day. It allows me to live a life full of possibilities I have not explored, and plenty to share with anyone who needs. Gifts abound.

This option is available to you as well, and it is *free*. Abundant thoughts bring abundance. Abound in love, and love bounces back to you. Think of good things, and they will come to visit you. Have you experienced thinking of someone you love, and they call you on the phone at that instant? The Universe responds, and it responds quickly. How wonderful is that? The Universe always provides. Fear, and perseveration on what you might lose, ensures only that the loss will occur. In the end, you are what you think. You can choose how you think by simply reconfiguring your desires for positive thoughts and positive emotions. Simply think LOVE. Indeed, love changes everything.

Manifesting intentions

With the preceding in mind, what are you going to do . . . *now*? Hypnotherapy is a wonderful experience, but you can start to put your own house in order while waiting for the maid to arrive.

Begin by determining what it is you want to change in your life. If you are facing something that seems overwhelming at the moment, break it into several smaller pieces. Start to make an initial plan for change.

Send an intention out to the Universe related to that change. Make it an affirmation. "This is what I want!" as opposed to "This is what I don't want." Make it specific, yet realistic. "I want to feel comfortable in my clothes;" "I want to experience joy in my work;" or "I want a life partner who is supportive and expresses love towards me" as opposed to "I want to lose forty pounds in the next three weeks;" "I want a big promotion and the corner office;" or "I'd like my spouse to drop dead."

Adopt language and behaviors consistent with that change. "I feel better in my clothes this week than I did two weeks ago" as opposed to "I only need to lose thirty more pounds and I'll feel good in my clothes." "This week's challenges at work give me an opportunity to demonstrate my skills and abilities" as opposed to "This week's tasks are demeaning to someone of my skills and abilities." "I acknowledge my error in selecting this spouse and will separate with maturity and responsibility" as opposed to "This relationship has tainted me for life."

To many, the positive intentions and language sound like Pollyanna. That's not the intent. If you want to create positive changes in your life, you have to prepare by conducting yourself in a fashion consistent with those changes. The positive energy within intentions and affirmative self-talk gradually accumulates, slowly changing scripts in your subconscious. Another way to look at it is that you behave positively long enough for the subconscious to adopt that mindset as its new script. It is a slower process than hypnotherapy, but it has the same effect over time. Repeated self-affirmations are a form of self-hypnosis that continually makes suggestions to the subconscious. When you eventually find yourself ready for hypnotherapy, it will be that much easier to accommodate the suggestions and recommendations of the therapist.

All hypnosis is self-hypnosis. Remember it is not about whether or not you can be hypnotized, it is really a matter of whether you wish to be. Unless you have an organic brain issue, you have the capacity to engage in trance work. The real question is whether or not you WANT to.

Our lives are manifestations of our imaginations. Good luck begins with good thoughts. It is all about how we mind our thoughts and how we go about setting our intentions. Sometimes we cannot always do for ourselves. We do better if people pray for us or even wish us luck. Get a little help. If self-hypnosis is not yet available to you, get an expert to help. Hypnotherapy is painless, and there are no drugs or pills to take. It is so simple that many people are suspicious of whether the process works. What can I say? I know I have changed the lives of many through my practice of hypnotherapy, but you don't have to take my word for it. If you are really curious, find a reputable hypnotherapist, check it out for yourself—you will be amazed!

EPILOGUE

I hope you have enjoyed your journey with me to discover an alternative path to attaining health and happiness. It took me many years of exploring a variety of disciplines to get to this tool. Are you willing to try it for your own healing?

In my studies related to hypnotherapy, I have learned a very important lesson.

All healing is spiritual work. Hypnotherapy is an incredibly effective tool in that work. If you trust it, and yourself, you can be transformed.

CHECKLIST

Do you:

   . . . feel that life is controlling you?
   . . . say yes when you want to say no?
   . . . feel that people are always judging you?
   . . . act in ways that are harmful to you?
   . . . wish to be more successful, accomplished or effective?
   . . . want to be loved?
   . . . feel undervalued, disrespected?
   . . . abuse food, cigarettes, drugs, alcohol, time or people?
   . . . have problems sleeping or staying focused?
   . . . have performance anxiety?
   . . . desire a life better than now?

If you answer yes to any of these, you can benefit from Integrative Hypnotherapy (IHT). This unique process helps you attain your goals by incorporating Clinical Hypnotherapy to facilitate changes you desire, Life Enhancement Training to teach you skills to sustain your changes, and Feng Shui principles to create environments that support your new desired behaviors.

For help or more information, contact:

iHealth Center for Integrated Wellness
     301 Main Street
     Roanoke, TX 76262
     Phone: 817-491-9809
     Email: *ihealthcenter@att.net*
     URL: *www.ihealththerapies.com*

BIBLIOGRAPHY

Here are some readings that are relevant to my studies in hypnotherapy and energy medicine. I hope you will find them helpful.

Achterberg, Jean. *Lightning at the Gate. A Visionary Journey of Healing*. Boston: Shambala Publications, 2002.

Achterberg, Jeanne, Barabara Dossey and Leslie Kolkmeier. *Rituals of Healing: Using Imagery for Health and Wellness*. New York: Bantam, 1994.

Acosta, Judith and Judith Prager. *The Worst is Over: What to Say When Every Moment Counts*. San Diego: Jodere Group, 2001.

Autry, James & Stephen Mitchell. *Real Power: Business Lessons from the Tao Te Ching*. New York: Riverhead, 1998.

Ballentine, Rudolph. *Radical Healing: Integrating the World's Great Therapeutic Traditions to Create a New Transformative Medicine*. New York: Crown Publishers, 1999.

Becker, Robert, and Gary Selden. *Body Electric. Electromagnetism and the Foundation of Life*. New York: Quill, 1985.

Beinfield, Harriet, & Efrem Krongold. *Between Heaven and Earth: A Guide to Chinese Medicine*. New York: Ballentine Wellspring, 1991.

Bender, Sue. *Everyday Sacred: A Woman's Journey Home*. New York: Harper Collins, 1999.

Bentov, Itzhak. *Stalking the Wild Pendulum: On the Mechanics of Consciousness*. Rochester, VT: Destiny, 1988.

Berliner, Helen. *Enlightened By Design: Using Contemplative Wisdom to Bring Peace, Wealth, Warmth & Energy Into Your Home*. Boston & London: Shambala, 1999.

Blok, Frits. *I Ching: Landscapes of the Soul: Revisiting an Ancient Chinese Oracle*. Amsterdam: Blozo Products Amsterdam, 2000.

Borysenko, Joan. *A Woman's Book of Life: The Biology, Psychology and Spirituality of the Feminine Life Cycle*. New York: Riverhead, 1996.

Boyne, Gil. *How to Teach Self-Hypnosis. Training Manual*. Glendale, CA: Hypnotism Training Institute of Los Angeles, 1987.

Boyne, Gil. *Transforming Therapy: A New Approach to Hypnotherapy*. Glendale, CA: Hypnotism Training Institute of Los Angeles, 1989.

Boyne, Gil. *Gil Boyne's Professional Hypnotism Training Course* (Manual). Glendale, CA: Hypnotism Training Institute of Los Angeles. 1991.

Brennan, Barbara. *Hands of Light: A Guide to Healing Through the Human Energy Field*. New York: Bantam New Age, 1988.

Brennan, Barbara. *Light Emerging: The Journey of Personal Healing*. New York: Bantam New Age, 1993.

Brennan, Margaret, and Merton Gill. *Hypnotherapy: A Survey of the Literature*. New York: John Wiley & Sons, 1964.

Bridges, Carol. *Soul in Place: Reclaiming Home as Sacred Space*. Nashville, IN: Earth Nation Publishing, 1995.

Bridges, Carol. *Code of the Goddess: Sacred Earth Feng Shui Oracle*. Nashville, IN: Earth Nation Publishing, 2001.

Bruyere, Rosalyn. *Wheels of Light: Chakras, Auras, and the Healing Energy of the Body*. New York: Fireside, 1994.

Buzan, Tony. *Mind Map Book: How to use Radiant Thinking to Maximize your Brain's Untapped Potential*. New York: Plume, 1993.

Chopra, Deepak. *Quantum Healing: Exploring the Frontiers of Mind/Body Medicine*. New York: Bantam, 1989.

Chopra, Deepak. *Path to Love: Renewing the Power of Spirit in Your Life*. New York: Harmony, 1997.

Chopra, Deepak. *How to Know God: The Soul's Journey into the Mysteries of Mysteries*. New York: Harmony, 2000.

Churchill, Randal. *Become the Dream: The Transforming Power of Hypnotic Dreamwork*. Santa Rosa, CA: Transforming Press, 1997.

Churchill, Randal. *Regression Hypnotherapy: Transcripts of Transformation*. Santa Rosa, CA: Transforming Press, 2002.

Cohen, Kenneth. *Way of Qigong: The Art and Science of Chinese Energy Healing*. New York: Ballantine, 1997.

Cousins, Norman. *Anatomy of an Illness as Perceived by the Patient*. New York: Bantam, 1979.

Dalai Lama. *Art of Living. A Guide to Contentment, Joy, and Fulfillment*. London: Thorsons, 2001.

Dalai Lama. *An Open Heart: Practicing Compassion in Everyday Life*. Boston: Little Brown & Company, 2001.

Dalai Lama, and Howard Cutler. *Art of Happiness: A Handbook for Living*. New York: Riverhead, 1998.

Dossey, Larry. *Reinventing Medicine: Beyond Mind-Body to a New Era of Healing*. San Francisco: HarperCollins, 1999.

Eden, Donna, and David Feinstein. *Energy Medicine*. New York: Jeremy Tarcher/Putnam, 1998.

Elman, Dave. *Hypnotherapy*. Glendale, CA: Westwood Publishing, 1964.

Emoto, Masaru. *Hidden Messages of Water*. New York: Atria, 2001

Emoto, Masaru. *True Power of Water: Healing and Discovering Ourselves*. New York: Atria, 2003.

Erickson, Milton. *Healing in Hypnosis*. New York: Irvington Publishers, 1983.

Feinstein, David, Donna Eden, and Gary Craig. *Promise of Energy Psychology*. New York: Penguin, 2005.

Fontana, David. *Secret Language of Dreams. Visual Key to Dreams and Their Meanings*. San Francisco: Chronicle, 1994.

Forrest, Derek. *Hypnotism: A History*. London: Penguin, 1999.

Fricker, Janert, and John Butler. *Secrets of Hypnotherapy*. London: Dorling Kindersley, 2001.

Gellatly, Angus, and Oscar Zarate. *Introducing Mind and Brain*. London: Totem, 1988.

Gerber, Richard. *Vibrational Medicine*. Rochester, VT: Bear & Company, 2001.

Gerber, Richard. *Practical Guide to Vibrational Medicine: Energy Healing and Spiritual Transformation*. New York: Quill, 2001.

Gordon, Richard. *Quantum-Touch: The Power to Heal*. Berkeley, CA: North Atlantic Books, 2002.

Gordon, Richard. *Your Healing Hands: The Polarity Experience*. Berkeley, CA: North Atlantic Books, 2004.

Harris, Gail. *Body & Soul: Your Guide to Health, Happiness and Total Well-Being*. New York: Kensington, 1998.

Hathaway, Michael. *Complete Idiot's Guide to Past Life Regression*. Indianapolis: Alpha, 2003.

Hay, Louise. *You Can Heal Yourself*. Carson, CA: Hay House, 1987.

Hahn, Thick Nhat. *Creating True Peace*. New York: Free Press, 2003.

Hawkins, David. *The Eye of the I: From Which Nothing is Hidden*. West Sedona, AZ: Veritas, 2001.

Hawkins, David. *Power vs. Force: The Hidden Determinants of Human Behavior* Carlsbad, CA: Hay House, 2002.

Hawkins, David. *I: Reality and Subjectivity*. West Sedona, AZ: Veritas, 2003.

Hewitt, William. *Truth About Hypnosis*. St. Paul, MN: Llewellyn Publications, 1996.

Houston, Jean. *Possible Human: A Course in Enhancing Your Physical, Mental and Creative Abilities*. Los Angeles: JP Tarcher, 1982.

Houston, Jean. *Life Force: The Psycho-Historical Recovery of the Self*. Madras, India/London: Quest, 1993.

Houston, Jean. *Mythic Life: Learning to Live our Greater Story*. San Francisco: Harper, 1996.

Houston, Jean. *Passion for the Possible: A Guide to Realizing Your True Potential*. San Francisco: Harper, 1997.

Hunt, Valeria. *Infinite Mind: Science of the Human Vibrations of Consciousness*. Malibu, CA: Malibu Publishing, 1996.

Ingerman, Sandra. *Medicine for the Earth*. Camarillo, CA: DeVorss, 1994.

Johnson, Robert. *Using Dreams and Active Imagination for Personal Growth*. San Francisco: HarperOne, 1989.

Karren, Keith, Brent Hafen, Lee Smith, and Katherine Frandsen. *Mind/Body Health: The Effect of Attitudes, Emotions, and Relationships*. San Francisco: Benjamin Cummings, 2002.

Koh, David. *Power of Geomancy*. Bandar Utama, Malaysia: Malaysian Institute of Geomancy Sciences, (n.d.).

Kuhn, Aihan. *Natural Healing with Qigong*. Boston: YMAA Publication Center, 2004.

Lam, Kam Kuen. *Chi Kung: The Way of Healing*. London: Gaia Books, 1999.

Lilly, Sue, and Simon Lilly. *Healing with Crystals and Chakra Energies*. London: Annes Publishing, 2005.

Lipton, Bruce. *Biology of Belief: Unleashing the Power of Consciousness, Matter and Miracles*. Santa Rosa, CA: Mountain of Love/Elite Books, 2005.

McGill, Ormond. *Professional Stage Hypnotism*. Glendale, CA: Westwood Publishing, 1977.

McGill, Ormond. *Hypnotism and Mysticism of India*. Glendale, CA: Westwood Publishing, 1979.

McGill, Ormond. *Hypnotism & Meditation: The Operational Manual to Hypnomeditation*. Glendale, CA: Westwood Publishing, 1981.

McGill, Ormond. *Seeing the Unseen: A Past Life Regression Revealed Through Hypnotic Regression*. Wales, UK: Crown Publishing, 1997.

McGill, Ormond. *Secrets of Dr. Zomb: The Autobiograpy of Ormond McGill*. Williston, VT: Crown House Publishing, 2003.

Minirth, Frank, Paul Meier, Robert Hemfelt, and Sharon Sneed. *Love Hunger: Recovery from Food Addiction*. Nashville, TN: Thomas Nelson Publishers, 1990.

Mukerjea, Dilip. *Braindancing: Brain-blazing Practical Techniques in Creativity for Immediate Application*. Singapore: Brainware Press, 2001.

Mukerjea, Dilip. *Surfing the Intellect*. Singapore: Brainware Press, 2001.

Myss, Carolyn. *Anatomy of the Spirit: The Seven Stages of Power and Healing*. New York: Random House, 1996.

Myss, Carolyn. *Scared Contracts: Awakening Your Divine Potential*. New York: Harmony, 2001.

Ody, Penelope. *Practical Chinese Medicine*. New York: Sterling Publishing, 2000.

Olness, Karen, and Gail Gardner. *Hypnosis and Hypnotherapy with Children*. Philadelphia: Gruene & Stratton, 1988.

Peck,Scott. *Road Less Traveled: The Unending Journey Toward Spiritual Growth*. New York: Simon & Shuster, 1993.

Peck, Scott. *Road Less Traveled & Beyond: Spiritual Growth in an Age of Anxiety*. New York: Simon & Shuster, 1997.

Peden, Laren. *I Ching: Discover the Ancient Chinese Art of Prophecy*. New York: Warner Books, 1996.

Pert, Candace. *Molecules of Emotion: The Science Behind Mind-Body Medicine*. New York: Touchstone, Simon & Shuster, 1997.

Pelletier, Kenneth. *Best Alternative Medicine*. New York: Simon & Shuster, 1999.

Prager, Judith. *Journey to Alternity: Transforming Healing Through Stories and Metaphors*. San Jose, CA: Writers Press Club, 2000.

Rossbach, Sarah. *Feng Shui: The Chinese Art of Placement*. New York: Penguin Compass, 2000.

Rossbach, Sarah, and Master Lin Yun. *Feng Shui Design: The Art of Creating Harmony for Interiors, Landscape and Architecture*. New York: Penguin Group, 1998.

Rossi, Ernest, and David Cheek. *Mind-Body Therapy: Methods of Ideodynamic Healing in Hypnosis*. New York: WW Norton & Company, 1988.

SantoPietro, Nancy. *Feng Shui and Health: The Anatomy of a Home: Using Feng Shui to Disarm Illness, Accelerate Recovery and Create Optimal Health*. New York: Three Rivers Press, 2002.

Sardello, Robert. *Freeing the Soul from Fear*. New York: Riverhead Books, 1999.

Schulz, Mona Lisa. *Awakening Intuition*. New York: Harmony, 1998.

Seaward, Brian. *Health of the Human Spirit: Spiritual Dimensions for Personal Health*. Needham Heights, MA: Allyn & Bacon, 2001.

Siegel, Bernie. *Love, Medicine, & Miracles: Lessons Learned about Self-Healing from a Surgeon's Experience with Exceptional Patients*. New York: Harper & Row, 1986.

Silvester, Trevor. *Wordweaving, Volume I: The Science of Suggestion: A Comprehensive Guide to Creating Hypnotic Language*. Chippenham, UK: Quest Institute, 2003.

Silvester, Trevor. *Wordweaving, Volume II: The Question is the Answer*. Burwell, Cambs/UK: Quest Institute, 2006.

Sylver, Marshall. *Passion, Profit & Power: Reprogram your Subconscious Mind to Create the Relationships, Wealth, and Well-Being that you Deserve*. New York: Simon & Shuster, 1995.

Thie, John, and Matthew Thie. *Touch for Health*. Camarillo, CA: DeVorss, 2005.

Tebbetts, Charles. *Self Hypnosis and Other Mind-Expanding Techniques*. Glendale, CA: Westwood Publishing, 1987.

Temes, Roberta. *Complete Idiot's Guide to Hypnosis*. Indianapolis, IN: Alpha Books, 2000.

Tutko, Thomas, and & Umberto Tosi. *Sports Psyching: Playing Your Best Game all of the Time*. New York: Jeremy Tarcher/Putnam, 1976.

Waterfield, Robin. *Story of Hypnosis*. London, UK: MacMillan, 2002.

Webster, Richard. *Art of Dowsing*. Edison, NJ: Castle Books, 1996.

Wolinshy, Stephen, H. *Way of the Human: The Quantum Psychology Notebooks, Volume 1*. Capitola, CA: Quantum Institute, 1999.

Yogananda, Paramahansa. *Autobiography of a Yogi*. Los Angeles: Self-Realization Fellowship, 2001.

Zukav, Gary. *Seat of the Soul*. New York: Simon & Shuster, 1990.

A SET OF BRIEF COMMENTS/SUMMARIES

Kweethai Neill's *Hypnotherapy: An Alternative Path to Health and Happiness* is a unique addition to the literature of hypnotherapy. This overview of the field is written in a personal, entertaining style that is friendly and engaging. Hypnotherapy is a very broad profession, and Dr. Neill takes advantage of her extensive experience to give a wide-ranging exploration that includes a special emphasis on health issues. Her excitement is contagious, and her insights and examples will give readers a deeper appreciation for the field.

—Randal Churchill, Director, Hypnotherapy Training Institute
Author, *Regression Hypnotherapy and Become the Dream*

Dr. Kweethai Neill is a highly skilled Hypnotherapist. Her new book *Hypnotherapy: An Alternative Path to Health and Happiness* is simply jam-packed with practical information and useful How To's in Hypnosis. Her experience is soon evident as you page through the chapters of the book. She provides the reader with a clear interpretation to otherwise complicated situations in easy-to-understand language. The information embraces the beginner as well as the seasoned professional. I recommend this book for anyone wanting to elicit healthy change in his/her life. Full of wisdom and self-help in all 17 chapters, the book has a place in every complementary wellness practitioner's library.

   —Robert F. Otto, PhD
     President and CEO
     The International Association of Counselors and Therapists
     The International Medical and Dental Hypnotherapy Association

After a successful academic career in health education, Kweethai Neill has turned her attention to the field of hypnotherapy and in this book she gives a clear and methodical account of hypnosis and the ways it can be used in therapy. Important principles of hypnotherapy are presented in an easily understandable manner for practitioners and public alike. Practical examples illustrate the theory and make it clear to the reader how hypnotherapy works in practice. This book is a particularly useful resource for the student seeking clarity and conciseness in a comprehensive review of the state of the art.

   —Dr. John Butler, principal instructor for the Hypnotherapy Training Institute of Britain
     Department of Anatomy & Human Science/Division of Reproduction & Endocrinology, King's College London School of Medicine

Perhaps you have always wondered about how your mind works, what really motivates you, how to make meaningful, healthful changes in your life. You know that 'willpower' alone, using your conscious mind, can take you only so far. If this is a subject you would like to know more about, *Hypnotherapy: An Alternative Path to Health & Happiness* is a good place to start. Kweethai Chin Neill has put together information, stories, and a great enthusiasm for the subject that will start you looking at your own processes differently, and once you do that, you are already on the path.

   —Judith Prager, PhD., author of *The Worst is Over: What to Say When Every Moment Counts and Journey to Alternity: Transforming Healing Through Stories and Metaphors.*

It can be said there are many roads and all paths lead up the mountain, but the path is easier when one follows a guide. It is entertaining, engrossing and enlightening to travel with Kweethai on her journey to a better life. Even better is the fact that she has left a rendering of how we can follow her and her journey to that life. It is my pleasure to recommend any therapist or seeker can gain much from adding this inspirational work to their library.

—Jerry Brandt, Hypnotherapist, Psychotherapist, NLP practitioner

Dr. Kweethai Neill is not only someone highly skilled in hypnotherapy, but also a health professional who is deeply devoted to her clients, students, and readers. Who she is and what she is all about are contained within the covers of this excellent book, *Hypnotherapy: An Alternative Path to Health and Happiness.* This is a concise, readable, user-friendly book on hypnotherapy that will inspire you to initiate personal behavior changes, equip you with practical skills to enhance your health and happiness, by setting you on an exciting personal path to self discovery. Be forewarned: Do not read this book if you are not ready to make changes in your life.

—Chwee Lye Chng, PhD., FAAHB, Regents Professor, Department of Kinesiology, Health Promotion and Recreation, University of North Texas

Dr. Kweethai C. Neill has masterfully crafted *Hypnotherapy: An Alternative Path to Health and Happiness.* As an accomplished health educator, she blends practical information with theories and best practices. This text is useful for both therapists and individuals desiring to become their best.

The text is enjoyable reading as it contains personal illustrations and insights into the author and her passion to help others on their journey to health and happiness, as she has created her own path. Her background in health education is the foundation for this useful information related to motivation for change, behavior changes and outcomes, and adherence after initial change. Read, change, and become your best!

—Jean Keller, Dean, College of Education, University of North Texas

ABOUT THE AUTHOR

After a successful career as a university professor, Dr. Kweethai Neill is a recovered academic. She left the halls of the university to embrace the Universe-city. As a child in Malaysia she aspired to become a brain surgeon. Now a health educator and hypnotherapist she changes minds, only she doesn't use a scalpel. She has expanded her focus from Mind-Body health to include and focus on Spirit, striving for a truly holistic approach to health and well-being. Dr. Neill is founder and president of the iHealth Center for Integrated Wellness, located in Roanoke, Texas.

Contact Dr. Neill at:

iHealth Center for Integrated Wellness
301 Main Street
Roanoke, Texas   76262

Phone: 817-491-9809
Email: *ihealthcenter@att.net*
URL: *www.ihealththerapies.com*

Thank you for reading this book. We would love to hear from you. Email us if you have any questions or comments.

If you are interested in becoming an exceptional clinical hypnotherapist or you are already in practice and wish to continue outstanding professional study with Dr. Kweethai and faculty at our school, please contact us below:

iHealth Hypnotherapy School
301 Main Street
Roanoke, Texas 76262
URL: www.ihealththerapies.com
E Mail : ihealthcenter@att.net
Phone: 817-491-9809

If you are interested in consulting Dr. Kweethai for private sessions or want her to come to your facility or event to deliver a seminar or keynote, please contact us below:

iHealth Center for Integrated Wellness Inc.
301 Main Street
Roanoke, Texas 76262
URL: www.ihealththerapies.com
E Mail : ihealthcenter@att.net
Phone: 817-491-9809

If you are interested in purchasing more copies of this book for your friends or students, please contact us below. If you are a school or would like to be a reseller, please make sure you ask for wholesale privileges.
Contact:

Dr. Steve Stork, Publications Director
301 Main Street
Roanoke, Texas 76262
URL: www.ihealththerapies.com
E Mail : ihealthcenter@att.net
Phone: 817-491-9809